I Left My Fat Behind

I Left My Fat Behind

By Barbara Zara

With Erin McHugh

A Stonesong Press Book

NEW CENTURY PUBLISHERS, INC.

Printing Code
12   13   14   15   16

Library of Congress Cataloging in Publication Data

Zara, Barbara.
  I left my fat behind.

  Includes index.
  1. Reducing diets. 2. Reducing diets—Recipes.
I. Title. RM222.2.Z364   613.2′5   82-2148
ISBN 0-8329-0122-9   AACR2

Printed in the United States of America

To

W.W.D.

Who will never see me with a fat behind.

Contents

Appendix

Foreword

This is not another diet book. It's a book about living the best life you can for yourself and loving the most important person around you—you. The ingredients here are self-esteem and some stamina. Together, we're going to make a new, slim you!

Do you want to lose weight? Now hold on a minute, don't answer so quickly. I'm not asking if you want to be instantly thin. I'm not asking if you wish it would fall off by morning. I'm asking if you *want* to be slim. Do you believe with all your heart it's possible? Are you willing to work toward that end? Then, and only then, will it happen. That's no idle promise from me, it's a fact.

No one wakes up in the morning and decides to get fat and it's not something that happens to us like a heart attack. It's a choice. We *choose* to overeat and hence have chosen to be fat. We've learned excuses that keep us obese. "I can't help it—I have no willpower." What is willpower? Have you ever seen it, touched it, tasted it? "I used to have willpower," you might say. Well, what happened to it? Did it pack its bags in the middle of the night and leave? Why is it that when we use the word willpower it's always to mention that we don't have any?

What we should be talking about is *want* power. If you want to be slim and happy, you can be. Every function of your body is controlled by your mind. Once you've planted that idea in your subconscious, it's plugged into that data bank until you take it out. Now, if you replace the idea that's in there now about how you're fat and there's nothing you can do about it with the positive idea that you can shed the unwanted pounds, your body will react to its new, positive programming.

How do I know? I've been there. I've got a degree in Binging from the Grand Union. And who is better qualified to help you lose weight than someone who knows all your tricks and bad habits? That's not something you learn in med school—they teach it in the cookie and candy section of your local supermarket.

I know exactly how you're feeling at this moment. I know the pain of obesity. I know the hurt that has been inflicted on you, and worse I know the hatred you have felt toward yourself. All this can change for you *now*, starting today, if you *believe* you can lose weight. *Fat cannot exist in your life unless you are willing to tolerate it.*

I'm 49 years old and I can truthfully say that I wasted 35 of those years. Not so long ago I weighed 211 pounds and was a candidate for the most miserable person in North America. I had tried all the gimmicks in the world, every fad diet, every low-cal cookie, special belts and peddlers and sauna suits. I had a dead-end job because my appearance made my chances for promotion negligible. My self-image was going to pieces and every morning I woke up thinking how awful it was going to be to have to go through another day of being Barbara Zara.

With the state I was in, it was pretty devastating to find out that *I* was the only one who could help me. But strength builds and I quickly learned that it was Barbara Zara who was going to help me out of my fat funk. And if I do say so myself, I did a hell of a good job.

I've written this book for one reason and one reason only: So that I can help as many people as possible enjoy the exciting and rewarding parts of life that they are now missing because they are depressed about being overweight.

As I said at the outset, this is not really a diet book, but a book about living up to your fullest expectations and being in control. And this book will work for you if you allow it to. There is no need for you to suffer as long as I did. You can make your own choices now and be happy and confident about them.

Throughout most of my life I tried to find a reason for my compulsive eating. I knew that a completely happy person doesn't punish oneself by becoming obese. Okay then, what is happiness? There are as many answers to that question as there are people asking it. There's my answer and your answer, but there is not *the* answer. To me, happiness is being in control. Not controlling others, but controlling my own life—that's enough to handle! I had spent years giving control away to people and things and then finding out I didn't like being run around like a robot. The result? Mutiny, every time. And in the fat world, mutiny is spelled E–A–T.

Life is an attitude and if you think and act like a winner, you'll be a winner. Believe it or not, we choose to be fat. We work hard for the privilege, staying up all night eating, getting up early in the morning so we can start again. Now we have to put in just as much time and effort into becoming slim. Change your attitude, believe in yourself. You're some-one important, one of a kind. You'll never be duplicated on the face of this earth. The only thing standing in the way of your success is you.

Nothing can exist in your life unless you are willing to tolerate it. If, starting today, you will no longer tolerate fat, it will be gone from your life. You and I have tolerated fat—in fact, we've invited it. There's no fat fairy who comes to our house in the middle of the night with a huge spatula that spreads fat all over us. We do it ourselves.

There's nothing you can do about yesterday. All your crying, guilt and wishing it were different can't change anything. It's history. But today, ah, that's where the magic is. Starting today you can change all the things in your life that need changing. Don't look back at yesterday as a failure. Look at it as a learning experience for a better today. You should enjoy every day as a child does.

You know, there's nothing wrong with being childlike. Even today, people still say to me, "Aren't you ever going to grow up?" Hey folks, if you haven't noticed, this is it—as up as I'm getting. Do they mean, "act my age"? Okay, what's a 49-year-old woman supposed to act like? Should I wear support stockings and orthopedic shoes? Put out a manual so I know what's expected of me.

Even after fourteen years of being slim, I still turn sideways and look at myself in the mirror every single morning. "Nothing succeeds like success" they say; there's a lot of truth in that. I find that I'm much more appreciative of everything now. I really enjoy the foods I eat because I take the time to savor each bite. I love being able to run if I have to catch a train. Slim, that is *always* slim, people just can't understand this. Everything is truly rosier for me.

Following my weight loss I started a group called Slim-U. As I left the house for my first meeting, I can remember thinking, "If only five people come tonight, I can build a group from there." I was so excited—I had so many things to tell my new members. I understood just what they were going through.

On that night, when I'd finished weighing everyone in, I walked to the front of the room, turned and looked at everyone and thought, "What in hell am I doing here?" If there had been some way I could have pulled a disappearing act at that moment, I would have. I was truly filled with absolute terror—my eyes were filling up with tears and my hands were cold and shaking. But one woman was looking me straight in the eye. She was very heavy and suddenly I realized that she was there because I had promised to help her. And I knew that I could.

Since that evening I've stood before a weight-loss group somewhere in the neighborhood of four thousand times and since our first group of 28 unhappy, overweight people walked into that room in Fort Lauderdale, my directors and I have helped thousands of people like yourselves lose literally millions of pounds.

Every meeting is as exciting to me as the first and I love to watch the expressions on those faces turn from doubtful, unhappy frowns to confident, happy smiles.

In *I Left My Fat Behind* you will read about people like yourself and people who've had an even worse time than you. (I know it's hard to imagine.) You will read about familiar situations and realize that you are not alone; you will howl with laughter at some of the things you and others have tried to pull off for the sake of food; you will come to know people like my friend Susan, who had no self-esteem and faced a bleak-looking future. Susan has lost a not-to-be-taken-lightly 260 pounds and is a prime mover at Slim-U.

I will teach you effective ways of dealing with your fat— and your fears. No tools or gimmicks—just a mixture of self confidence, control and common sense. You'll find that your own best friend is not a cheesecake, but you!

It's really not too painful. In fact, there's nothing more satisfying than finding that you are the one controlling your diet instead of a protein drink made of bean sprouts. If you're honest with yourself and follow the ideas set forth in these pages and use some of the recipes here instead of the more fattening ones you're using now, I personally guarantee you those pounds of fat will start to disappear. Don't be surprised—it's no big promise, just a fact. Maybe this book will make you cry a little, hopefully it will make you laugh a lot, but if we go through it together, it's going to work. *I* believe in you and I don't even *know* you. But if you truly believe you can lose weight, you will. And you'll keep it off forever.

Remember that any weight reduction program should have your doctor's approval. Consult with your physician before starting your own or any other diet plan.

Unfortunately, I'll never meet most of the people who will read this book. But if I did meet you I would tell you that you can be as successful as you believe you can be. I wasn't born a winner. I chose to be one. I worked at it. I can't give you any miracle cures—but I can help you see that you're worth more than anyone else in the world.

So let's start *now.* I can't wait to meet the new slim you— and I bet you can't either.

ONE

The Not-So-Good Old Days

1

Deep Throat—How My Career Began

OK, pal, drop it. NOW. That's right. Now that you've settled in with some cookies and hot chocolate to read the incredible thriller of how Barbara Zara lost 90 pounds and then went on to help others (you're next) lose over a million, I want you to get that trigger finger off the goods. No more peanut butter, French fries, candy. Tomorrow is not the time to start losing weight. There's always a tomorrow, always another Monday to start a new diet. And if you've gone out and spent the money to find out how *I Left My Fat Behind*, you're probably pretty serious about losing weight. So start *now*. I promise to help you if you wipe all that chocolate off of your sticky fingers.

I Left My Fat Behind is the true story of how I fought my personal Battle of the Bulge—and won. Believe me, it was no Six-Day War either. It wasn't easy, but my final successful skirmish led me to several convictions: not only was I infinitely happier and more attractive, the new me felt so good and positive that I suddenly had a missionary's zeal to convert others. I knew that if the Peanut Butter Queen of Succasunna, New Jersey could go straight, anyone could. After thirty years in Lard Limbo, the energy and self-confidence that I had gained from my triumph led me to start my own weight loss groups. I wanted to spread the word—and help others reduce the spread. And like I said—you're next.

This book is a distillation of all I learned from my struggles and the struggles of all my friends at Slim-U. Let's not call it a diet book—there isn't an overweight person in America who doesn't know what *not* to eat. It's a book about *you*—because, let's face it, it ain't the Twinkies that are making you fat—it's you. It's your attitudes, self-perception and bad habits that are keeping you fat. It's *you* who's keeping you fat. This book is about choice. Your choice to be a Slim Somebody rather than a big fat nobody. If you will expend 25% of the energy you put into getting fat into making the right choices for yourself, you'll be slim in no time at all. So how about it?

I promised to help you—but I can't promise you'll lose weight. You'll have to make—and keep—that promise to yourself. Would that I could jump out of these pages and hug you for not sticking your pudgy hand into a candy dish—but I can't. But together we can explore and solve the problems and change the behavior that have made you overweight. I'll show you how, with encouragement, examples, a lot of laughter—and maybe a few tears. You'll find yourself pounds lighter and infinitely more lighthearted. I am asking you to change your life for your own good, mentally and physically. Believe me, you're worth it. I know, I did it myself, and the silver #1 I wear around my neck says it all. Now it's your turn.

In the Beginning

When I presented myself to my mother, I was a squalling, red-faced bundle of joy and healthiness. The pink satin baby book I still treasure tells the tale of my precocious growth.

> Barbara is a very good eater and always finishes everything on her plate. Her favorite foods are potatoes, cookies and bread with peanut butter and jelly.

And you wonder how an adorable little 7 lb. 3 oz. baby becomes a 211-lb. lady? Look back and remember for yourselves ...

I'll bet you learned before you could talk, as I did, that if you were well-behaved you got a reward. We all know what form that reward took—food. "Let mommy finish her housework in peace and I'll make you a nice peanut butter and marshmallow sandwich." "You've had a long day at school—how about some brownies and milk?" And we still do it today. "I worked like a dog all morning; I think I'll treat myself to a salami hero for lunch." It would be quite an understatement to say it adds up. By the time I was sixteen, I weighed 185, and the squalling had turned to tears of anger and frustration: tears that stayed with me a long time, even though I learned to put up a good front and to turn the pain inside out into laughter. Remember the Christmas those reindeer sweaters were popular? My sister and I each got one. They delicately pranced across her chest, while mine looked as if they were climbing the Alps. I grew out of it before they ever reached the top.

But it wasn't till I was 35—and weighed 211—that I finally came to my senses. I kept telling myself that gaining 26 pounds in 26 years was a terrific track record. Terrific until the day I ran my pudgy hand down a doctor's ideal weight–height chart. I discovered that if I were a 6′2″ man with a heavy frame, I'd still be six pounds overweight. Then it sunk in that maybe I had to lose a little more than six pounds—in fact, a little more than 90! I panicked. But right then and there I did the most difficult thing I have ever done: admitted to myself that I was obese and that I hated it. Hated it!

Well, I had spent 35 years working at getting fat. I realized the job had been an enormous success. If I had gotten paid for all the work I put into it, I'd be a millionaire. They say you can never be too rich or too thin, and I was neither. I was sick of saying "I have nothing to wear", when the truth was that I had a closet full of clothes in sizes 16 to 22½, testifying to various failures at dieting. I was fed up with being jolly because everyone *said* fat people are jolly. I'd had it.

Taking the Plunge

Shakily, I called one of my closest friends, an ex-fatty who had dropped 45 pounds and was looking—and acting— like Eileen Ford's top model. She gave me the number of the weight loss group she had joined, but it still took me three weeks to convince myself that I was truly committed to change. That decision—made *by* me, *for* me—improved my life more than any other decision I've ever made.

I learned the two major factors you need to be aware of to lose weight: self-love and the desire to change.

The pounds didn't melt away magically, but the love and encouragement I received, and my ultimate satisfaction at reaching my goal made the struggle well worth the effort. Along the way, I learned a thing or two about myself, about the real pain we hide behind our smiles, about the fears and destructive feelings I had been feeding right along with my face as I stuffed it with candy, cookies and junk food. The self-confidence and control I gained are two things I wouldn't give up for all the chocolate cake in the world.

Let me give you a few well-researched words about diets—and I know, I've tried them all. Any program that promises you quick weight loss is useless. I've lost 25 pounds 25 times. It took me that long to realize I was a yo-yo in more ways than one—and that the fattest thing about me was my head.

When I finally faced myself (and there was a lot to be faced!), I realized that all of the diets had one thing in common: *they took the responsibility for weight loss away from me.* These diets were running *me*, I wasn't running *them*, and I was going around in circles. Relinquishing control seems like a swell idea, but it's what makes those diets useless in the long run, because when you go off them, you *still* don't have any control. You know the regimes I mean: the barely legible photocopied page from a friend at the office who swears he's tried it and lost 37 pounds (only he doesn't say he gains back three a week). These diets tell you what, when, how, what color, and what kind of fork to use. But these plans create two large problems (to add to the huge one you already have): physiological imbalance and mental dependency. They leave you bored and regimented. You'll lose weight for a while—but you won't have the satisfaction of tackling and conquering the problem because you've been on automatic pilot.

The diet is a success, not you. When the tyranny of tea and toast is over, you jump at the reward of macaroni and beers and the scales jump right along with you. The big reward? A closetful of clothes that are too small and a rapidly increasing waistline. Not to mention a king-sized case of the guilts.

Nothing is so important in losing weight as the self-esteem you are gaining from controlling your own life.

You know, we fatties really do work at getting fat. Just think about it. You stay up late to sneak snacks, get up early so you can have your breakfast and some of the kids', too. You spend limitless mental effort on lies and excuses: I haven't eaten all day (except standing up in front of the refrigerator, cramming yesterday's leftovers down your throat); just a little won't hurt (when have you ever been able to eat just a little?); if I don't mind myself this way, no one else should (but is that true?); I deserve it, or I *need* it. If you are like I was, food becomes your friend, lover, tranquilizer and reward. Have you ever noticed that thin people don't make excuses for eating, and fat ones do?

Well, it's time to stop. Right now, today. Put all of that effort you've put into making excuses into changing your life. Choose to be thin! "But I can't," you wail. There's a party tonight..." "It's my glands, nerves, genes..." You'll find an excuse. But there's no excuse for continuing to hate yourself. No matter how well you've been hiding it, show me a fat person and I'll show you a self-hater. Not convinced?

Consider this. Do you like (much less love) the fact that when you walk down the street, your rear end looks like two midgets wrestling under a blanket? Is your favorite fashion a polyester tunic whipped up by Omar the Tentmaker? Do you think heart attacks, high blood pressure, kidney failure, back problems and a lousy sex life happen only on *General Hospital*, or do you realize that they're very real threats to *your* health? If you've forgotten that you own a full-length mirror, if it's been six months since you sat in a man's lap and six months since you've seen same (if he's still in the land of the living after that experience), then you are a candidate for a new you.

How do you think you put on all that weight anyway? If you're like me, as I mentioned before, it started with plain old bribery from mom. And as a child, you were probably never called fat, at least not by grown-ups. A grown-up's world is full of euphemisms for kids they hope will lose weight—remember "Chubette" and "Husky" sizes? Nancy Drew's friend Bess who was "pleasingly plump"? Your parents chose to ignore the problem like you did, hoping it would just go away. Nobody wanted to admit it, but you were on your way to being a full-fledged fatty. Parents claim a fat child is a healthy child. And there was a lot of enforcement to eat and eat well. Remember the one-way guilt ticket to fat? "Eat those turnips! Just think of the starving children in Europe!" I'm convinced I saved an entire continent from malnutrition, yet I've never even gotten a thank-you note from Save the Children.

Health and beauty were excuses parents often used on you, too. "Eat all your crusts or you won't have curly hair." I even ate my sister's crusts, and I'm still in the bathroom every morning with the hot rollers. And if carrots are so great for your vision, how come I have to use magnifying glasses to read the "For Sale" column? And on and on. "Spinach will make you strong like Popeye! Liver gives you rich blood! An apple a day keeps the doctor away! Prunes make you regular! Milk makes your teeth healthy! Enjoy! Enjoy" Still enjoying it now?

After a lifetime of following these "health tips," needless to say I was in excess 90 pounds overweight and had developed a large case of self-loathing that was almost as hard to drag around as the rest of me.

Somewhere along the line (I don't know exactly where) food had ceased to be a pleasure and a nutritional requirement: it had become an obsession. Face it, what fatty eats out of hunger? You eat because you're bored, or nervous, or depressed (because you're so fat?), or to punish yourself, or simply because the food is there. But this is the most important thing to remember—mom's reward system may have started you on the road to Fatdom, but you waddled the rest of the way all by yourself. One tough lesson to learn is that when you start pointing the finger of blame, you've got to point it at yourself.

Making New Rules for Yourself

So how do you get off Fat Street? One of the first things you are going to have to learn is to accept responsibility for your own actions and discard all the rules and regulations you've acquired that are untrue, hurtful or useless. Throw out "I'm a failure" first. Just getting through an ordinary day is cause for celebration. Throw failure out of your vocabulary completely—it now no longer applies to dieting, love, parenting, sex, careers, housekeeping or any other aspect of your life.

Make your own rules and play by them. You'll come up a winner!

Does this all sound like too much? Starting to squirm? "But I don't have the willpower!" I can hear it now—it used to be one of my favorite excuses. Unfortunately, I couldn't find a six-pack of willpower in any of my local grocery stores. Forget willpower—what you need is the very real desire to change and improve yourself. And along the way there will be good days, and there will be lapses: the strawberry cheesecake that leaps down your throat before you can make a move to stop it, as if *it* were Bruce Jenner; the hot fudge sundae you "reward" yourself with that is calorically equal to the food a village in India eats in an entire week; the time you cheat and have meatballs and spaghetti and three beers for dinner. But consider this: what "reward" is there for being fat? Do you want to spend the rest of your time on this earth engaged in life and death struggles with your girdle, hiding from sales ladies and fellow customers in the dressing rooms of your favorite clothes store, and laughing at fat jokes that cut you to the quick? When you cheat, who are you cheating? Only the nice thin person lurking behind your mammoth exterior, longing to make an entrance clad in a clinging knit with no visible ripples and bulges.

I know you. I *was* you. I'm the lady who cleaned her house of all forbidden foods, gave the car keys to her husband so she couldn't drive to the supermarket, and in a funk, sent herself a candygram. I'm the one who attended weight loss groups, and begged a fellow fatty who had sinned to describe the chocolate cake that was her undoing "just one more time." Finally, though, I was the one who realized that I was simply miserable being fat, and that I had done it to myself, and that it was time to make myself happy.

But I'm also the lady who panicked at the idea of being slim: fear of the unknown can be a real force against losing weight. I'd lived with my fat self for a long time, as you probably have. If you're like me, you may think you feel comfortable the way you always have been. Don't mistake the familiar for the comfortable—change can be scary, but when it's for the better, it's the best high I know. Do you feel that you *are* fat, and that you might not be able to handle the demands of a slim and healthy person? That's scary, too, but the beauty of my program is that you gain confidence as you lose weight. Your payment is pounds lost, your payoff is lasting personality plusses. Becoming thin won't guarantee you a dashing Prince Charming, a high-paying new career or fabulously interesting friends. But if you stay the way you are, the chances of these things happening are often as slim as you are fat.

End of the Affair

If you choose to control your life, you'll improve it in more ways than just slimming down. It stands to reason that all the time you put into being obese—thinking about food, shopping for food, preparing it, eating it, feeling guilty about having consumed your way through another day (whew!)— all that time would be free. In the course of this book, I am going to show you how to live with your new-found time— how to enjoy it and get real pleasure from it—instead of killing it, working to feed your face.

We will also look honestly at how, when and why we eat—and eat and eat—and I think you'll be surprised. We'll explore the emotional lows of being fat and the unexpected side effects—good and bad—of losing weight. I'll help you learn, through Slim-U menus and eating plans, how to enjoy foods you never thought could have the orgasmic effect of a pizza. You're going to change your entire way of thinking about the world and your place in it—your new perceptions will not only help you lose weight, they will help you keep it off. Forever. Most of all, I am going to remind you of something that you've probably forgotten long ago—how to love yourself. By the time we are finished, you *will* have an enormous appetite—for life!

2

End of the Road

Believe me, there comes a day when you've finally had it. Maybe it's because the doctor almost scared you into that heart attack he's been promising for so long. Or maybe your daughter came home from school and mentioned that her teacher called you obese. Perhaps you're tired of black tent dresses. Or even because someone shook you hard enough to make you realize that there was a beautiful slim person inside that beautiful fat person. All these things happened to me. And after trying every diet known to fatkind, I decided to call my friend Edna, who had just joined a weight loss group.

I called Edna alright. In fact, I hung up on her three times before I worked up the courage to speak to her. I know as well as you do what it takes to call someone for the express purpose of saying "Hi, I'm fat. Please help me." It took me 20 minutes of inane questions before I finally had the nerve to ask the name of the group. Secretly I was overjoyed when Edna said the meetings were on Monday nights. I had called on a Tuesday, so I had six whole days till Death Row.

Well, if God made the world in six days, I sure as hell tried to match Him by *eating* it in the same amount of time. And just like God, on the seventh day I rested. You've got it— Monday night rolled around and I sat home because I had done myself in. I had eaten so much in the previous week and felt so guilty that I couldn't bear to cart my fat self to that meeting. So I gave myself a week's reprieve and started another eatathon.

But what of the famous Edna, and how was she faring on the scales? Either misery loves company or she was just a good soul, because Edna started to call, wondering why I had changed my mind, and I began to get scared. All the good hard work fatties put into excuses suddenly went into worrying. What if I'm truly mentally unbalanced, and I can't stay on this diet? What if I know people at the meeting and I flunk out? Even after almost fourteen years, I still cringe when I think of the hell I put myself through in those couple of weeks.

Finally I committed the cardinal sin of telling my husband, Bill, that I was joining a weight loss group. Worse yet, in my temporary state of insanity, I babbled when and where, too. All the important, well-kept secrets were out.

The Beginning of the End

From that moment on, Bill kept an eagle eye on every morsel I touched, warning me that I had better taper off a bit. Just what I needed. Here I was about to face the firing squad and I've got a heckler on the sidelines.

I can remember waking up that morning and looking out the upstairs window and thinking, Lord, it looks just like any ordinary day, there are people going to work just like any other Monday morning, kids leaving for school and sloshing through the fresh snow. Did anybody care what was going to happen to me that very night? Didn't anybody care?

That night I pulled into the parking lot and saw a few cars I recognized, but I was frozen to my seat. I thought I'd give myself a lift by watching some of the other porkos waddle in first.

However, I was mortified. I saw women breeze in there who had waistlines and I was heartbroken. If this is the type of woman who goes to weight groups, I thought, then where do the truly fat people like me go? In tears, I put my key back into the ignition as another car pulled up beside me. When I saw the driver trying to squeeze out from behind the wheel, I felt a little better. I'm afraid it's human nature to sometimes feel better after seing someone worse off than you. When I saw that poor woman make three tries before she managed to get out of that car, my heart went out to her. If I had thought about going home a minute ago, I now decided to stay.

I wasn't at all sure on that bitter cold night in Suc- casunna *how* I was going to shed all that fat I had clung to for all those years, but I did know I was tired of being obese. And that's all I needed. *I had the will to change.*

If you've ever joined a weight group, you know how I felt when I went into that first meeting. Automatically, you scan the room hoping to find someone a little fatter, or even just as fat, as you are.

When I first stepped on that scale, my group leader looked me in the eye and said, "You don't have to be fat." I was shocked. All my life I had heard, "Everybody loves you just the way you are." "You have such a great personality that no one cares about your weight." "You always look so neat." All these friends thought they were being nice, and they meant well. And frankly, for years I was grateful for their devotion and tact. But while they were telling me how swell I was, I misconstrued what that all meant. They were stroking me in different places, making up for my fatness. And for 35 years I treasured their compliments. Until my first weight loss meeting, when I learned the truth:

I had a choice!

Don't think for a minute that I wasn't scared right out of my size 22½ excuse for a dress. That choice is a huge responsibility. But it wasn't bigger than me. I *wanted* to change. My new fairy-godmother-cum-group-leader talked to all of us as if she were certain that we all could and would be slim. She started on our eating habits—no more sneaking food. Could she possibly mean that we would be eating in front of our families after I had spent over 35 years perfecting the art of camouflaged eating? Nevertheless, I was mesmerized and I left there feeling I would never lust for a Twinkie again.

Bill had a million questions, and I thought I had all the answers. Tomorrow morning, I would have one egg, one piece of toast and a cup of tea. For lunch, a large tossed salad and a piece of fruit. Dinner—fish, another salad, string beans and a baked apple. Before bed, we were allowed another fruit and a beverage. Bill was amazed that I could eat all that food and still lose weight. All that food? Little did he know that I usually ate that amount of food for lunch.

I could hardly sleep that night. I was on my way to being a new person and contemplating what thin people do with their lives. What could they possibly do while watching Johnny Carson, how do they make dinner without sampling half of what they're preparing, what do slim women wear instead of a girdle, what it would feel like to sit down and be able to cross my legs? So far, I was really enjoying my diet ...

The Longest Day

I actually did well at breakfast, savoring the healthiness of my premiere dietary meal, but without a break for cookies, it looked by ten o'clock as though lunchtime would never come. Promptly at 11:30 I began shredding a head of lettuce. Knowing I could eat as much salad as I wanted, I prepared a feast Peter Rabbit would have paid $75 a plate for. I can barely remember that meal, but it started at noon and ended at 12:05.

I managed to steer clear of the kitchen till it was time to start dinner at 4:30. Things went smoothly until I opened the refrigerator door, and there it was, my first real temptation: A walnut coffee cake. I knew I couldn't have any but I could feel myself sliding back to my old excuses. I was rooted to the kitchen floor.

What harm would it do if I were to just pick off a few walnuts? It's not the same as eating the cake. After all, when you've been successful on a diet all day, you're entitled to a little something. How many times have I removed all the nuts in the blink of an eye? It's better known in the fat world as neutering a coffee cake. First you remove the nuts as carefully as possible, then you wet a butter knife and swirl the icing over all the tiny brown holes. Now, of course, the box must go, because it just wouldn't do for the label to read "Walnut Delight" when all the walnuts are gone, and thus, most of the delight. I would slide the cake onto a plate, cover it with plastic wrap and no one would ever be the wiser.

I don't know how I managed to handle it, but the crisis passed. I put the lid back on the box and closed the door. I must have looked at that cake five more times while I made dinner. *But I didn't touch it.*

That's the way control, willpower, self-denial, whatever you want to call it, really works. A minute at a time. An alcoholic doesn't sit down and say, "I will *never* have a drink again in my life." Forever is a very long time, my friend, and no one, but no one, can take it on all at once. All an alcoholic, or a gambler, or an overweight person, can do is practice self-control a moment at a time.

Set goals for yourself—and don't reach too high. The euphoria I felt after my first meeting was obviously not strong enough to conquer my hunger the next day. But the pride I felt when I went to bed after my first full day of dieting far surpassed that dreamy euphoria of the previous night *because it was real*. I had accomplished something I had never done before. And I found on the next day, and the next, that I didn't say to myself "I won't cheat until Johnny Carson." I took it one moment at a time. I won't cheat before lunch, or I won't touch that piece of cake someone is offering me this very minute. Work on *now*. Say no now, and you'll undoubtedly say no again. *Carpe diem* goes the old Latin proverb—"seize the day." Well, seize each moment that you succeed in your lessons of self-control and gloat over them. Each time you win, you're congratulating the best friend you've got.

Encountering a Former Fatty—You!

Let me warn you about an obstacle you'll probably encounter—the old you. Wait till you've found out how much you've been lying about your eating habits over the years. Now would be the time to eat humble pie, if it were on your diet. Since it's not, 'fes up, because you're about to encounter your past.

For example—that fateful first day of my diet. Enter one slim husband, sniffing approvingly at the smells emanating from the kitchen. I ask you, how good can baked fish, cauliflower and tossed salad smell? Almost as good as it tastes when you haven't been stuffing your face full of junk all day.

My first instinct was to suck the food off my plate like a vacuum cleaner, but I drew a deep breath, picked up my fork and tried to eat slowly, the way thin people do. One bite at a time. At that rate it took me fifteen or twenty minutes to eat half the food I normally ate in five. I was aware of Bill staring at me with a look of disbelief. Then it hit me—this was probably the first time my family had ever seen me sit at the table for a meal. Usually I had eaten enough while preparing the meal so that I was free to serve and clear while they relaxed over dinner.

Your new habits are going to unsettle those around you—so be prepared. Just as you are about to burst with pride at your control (as I was at that dinner table) someone is bound to pipe up with "What kind of diet is this? I don't want to hurt your feelings, but it seems that you're eating more now than you did before you decided to cut down." In your state of shock, you will probably decide to do one of three things to said someone:

1. smile sweetly and continue eating slowly;
2. tell X the truth about where you've been hiding the Oh! Henry's all these years; or
3. flatten them.

My suggestion would be the second, but then, hindsight is always 20/20, and there's nothing like getting out your aggressions.

So, looks like all your cheating has backfired, eh? There will be many times no one will understand how rough your choice to be slim is on you. What passes for normality in eating in the slim world is just a good intention in fatdom. Take, for instance, the chocolate chip cookie episode that occured early on in my fight for slimness. In my eyes, I was the saint of the bakery world, a true humanitarian in offering to bake cookies for my family while I was dieting. There had been many times when two or three packages of dough have never made it to the oven in my kitchen, and only 30 or so out of several dozen complete the arduous journey from oven to cookie jar. But that day I was invincible. I lost myself in my work. Beating, whipping, striking out, ridding myself of all frustrations. And for the first time in my baking career, not one chip had jumped from the bag into my mouth. Not to mention the nearly impossible task of getting sticky cookie dough off the spatula onto the sheet without using my fingers. But I was actually shaking—I didn't think I was going to make it.

I yelled for my husband. "Bill, count the cookies."

"Why should I count cookies?" (Stupid question.)

"So you'll know if any are missing." (He doesn't know. He honestly doesn't know.)

He counted 22. "Says here it makes two dozen, so you must have had your two already."

Now I knew in my heart of hearts I hadn't so much as touched that batter with mortal hands, and here was someone who loved me, doubting me. I can see only now that his thoughts of a bit of cheating were normal—*for a slim person.* But I had been the little boy who cried wolf for so many years that my small victories meant nothing to anyone else. It was then that I realized I was fighting my own battle, and that no one cared so much about Barbara Zara getting thin as Barbara Zara did.

Applaud Yourself

If you weigh 211 pounds—or more, or less—as I did, there's no person alive, no matter how much they love you, who's going to be overjoyed when your weekly weigh-in touts that you've lost three pounds. Three pounds from 211 pounds doesn't spell victory to anyone else, and let's face it, won't be obvious to people who see you on the street. But while it's adding up, week by week, you're taking a weight off your shoulders and a load off your mind that Atlas couldn't handle. Why? Because you have chosen to take control of *you!*

You're not only improving yourself physically, you're improving your attitude about you—no one can stop someone who's physically *and* emotionally put his mind to something. *Don't let your weight control you any longer!* You know, you could cope with the most difficult situations imaginable.

We've all heard stories of mothers who can't swim rescuing a drowning child, men who've made financial empires out of nothing, husbands and wives who give their broken marriages one more chance and succeed. There are even more incredible tales than this, I'm certain. Stories of people who take control where they haven't before to save someone they love. Well, those who love you try to help. Maybe they don't go about it quite the right way, but their left-handed compliments come from their hearts. *But they can't help you lose weight.* Why don't you give them a hand in loving you? Who matters more than you?

TWO

Change Is Not a Nickel and a Dime

3

Getting Off the Bandwagon

One of the first things that will hit you when you realize that you've decided to tolerate fat for the last day in your life (which is *today*, if you've already forgotten) is "How am I ever going to change?" It's a pretty good question, to tell you the truth. Let's face it, you've put your heart, soul and big mouth into getting fat all these years. For many people, it's not the thought of no more eclairs that does them in, but "What will I do while I'm talking on the phone?" or "Who can play bridge without peanuts?" If you had put all the time and energy you've spent eating all these years to work, you would probably be pulling in an extra 50 G's for Uncle Sam to tax. But since you've been concentrating on food, it will be damn hard to get your mind off it.

Now this doesn't mean you have to give up playing bridge in order to stay on your diet—in fact, just the opposite. You've got to learn to cope with food being around you—because it will be, everywhere you go. If you think you just may possibly faint of starvation during your next Grand Slam, just take along some legal food of your own. Think about it—you're not really enjoying or concentrating on the food anyway if you've managed a Grand Slam. You're just reaching for something to put in your mouth out of habit. There's no need to be embarrassed about bringing your own food, either. Your friends will be impressed to see that you're making the effort, and will respect your wishes when they see that you truly don't want to be tempted. This time you're serious and your plate of unfattening food tells everyone right off that you're attempting what has now seemed super-human to you—getting thin.

Ridding Yourself of Bad Habits

But maybe that's not the kind of thing you're afraid of— perhaps you're just the kind of person who has an aversion to changing for changing's sake. If you find yourself saying more often than not "Why should I change? This is the way I've done it all my life," then you'll find yourself in for a big surprise, because there are a lot of things that have *got* to change if you're serious about losing weight. Do any of these situations apply to you?

- Do you think you eat a lot of real junk? Yeah, you know the stuff I mean, and if you said to yourself "Like what?" then you sure as hell do.
- Do you find yourself involved in some useless activities that you've unconsciously gotten into because they provide chances to eat?
- Do you hang around the kitchen a lot? Is there a TV in there? A phone? If you've got another phone in the

house, use it. That will save you a pound a week right there. Don't give yourself reasons to go into the kitchen when it's not mealtime.
- Do you think of yourself? If you automatically say yes, think again. Because if you were *really* thinking about yourself, you'd be thinking about your health, both physical and mental, about how much you really love bikinis, about how happy you'd be if you looked like *her*. Well, maybe she's not as happy as you think she is, but wouldn't you like to try it and see?

OK, OK, so those are just a few tips. But they lead to *change*, good change, because you're ridding yourself of bad habits. How you're going to change on the whole is manifested in little tricks like these, but the real basis for changing is going to be in your outlook towards yourself. And that all fits nicely into one skinny word here called control.

You will never succeed at anything if you're not in control.

Getting Your Life Back into Control

You may think you don't have an ounce of control left, but stop and think about how you manage to control aspects of your life each day and how, if you find you are not managing well, you attempt change.

If you realize you are tired every morning, you start going to bed earlier; if your workload at the office becomes heavier, you know how to adjust your schedule so that you can handle the extra work; if something is bothering you, you know enough to talk to someone who can help. All I'm saying is that people cope. Some better than others, but we do cope. Why is it then that when it comes to controlling our eating habits, we refuse to do so. That's right—*refuse*.

Think about the number of times in a day that you do manage to say no: to someone pushing magazine subscriptions, to the lure of a department store display, to the temptation of staying home from work. If you write them down you'll find you're much more in control than you ever imagined.

Basically, all I'm telling you is that you're only fooling yourself if you say you have no control—and you're doing it on purpose. You're doing it, you're saying it, because *you want someone else to control you.* Hold on now, don't get indignant. When it becomes convenient for us, we often pass the buck and let someone else take over. Even Ronnie Reagan throws up his hands every once in a while and says "Holy Moses, let someone *else* make this decision." Don't get me wrong—the President of the United States and you and I all like to take the responsibility when it's easy on us, but everyone likes the heat taken off now and then, or else they wouldn't have invented air-conditioning. But in the long run, you have to take control of yourself every day of your life. I've held down three jobs. I've been a bored employee, a wife and mother, and a corporation president. And I'll tell you something right now—they are all equally difficult, each with their own unique problems. And somehow I controlled them all—with some mistakes along the way, to be sure—but just by living day to day, trying like hell to be in control, never a speck "better" or more special than anyone else on this earth. That control got me from a miserable woman who was in a huge rut to someone who loves to get up every morning and take control of my future, whether it's an hour or years away. And that control, my friends, is what brought me from 211 pounds down to 121. It may not be easy, but the rewards are priceless.

Giving and Taking Control

You know, for years I thought my mother or husband or employer would take care of everything, take control. I was just like a yo-yo, swinging back and forth between my responsibilities. But I learned a funny thing—no one does it right for me except me. Sooner or later you'll find that you have to do it yourself—and then you wonder what took you so long.

Here's an example...

During one of our rap sessions at Slim-U retreat, Alice stated that although she seemed to be able to handle a great deal of pressure and stress, the one situation that would send her into an eating frenzy was spending time with her mother—even speaking to her on the phone seemed to cause Alice to inhale a package of cookies. "I know she doesn't upset me on purpose," moaned Alice, "in fact, I don't think she even realizes the impact she has on me. Let me tell you something that happened recently."

"I dearly loved my father and his recent death was a terrible blow to me. I decided that there were so many lovely things that my dad had done throughout his life that I would like to write his eulogy and read it at his funeral. I'm basically a very shy person, and for me to stand before my family and friends and read this was a real milestone for me. Later everyone complimented me and I felt very proud that I had paid this last tribute to my father. I was not prepared for my mother's reaction, however. She stalked right up to me and said 'I bet you won't write one for me when I'm gone because you always favored your father.'"

Needless to say, Alice was speechless and deeply crushed. At a time like that, the last thing anyone needs is to have a large load of guilt heaped on them. "As hard as I tried, I just couldn't take it, and I lost control," Alice told us. Ah, there's that phrase again. *I lost control.*

Wrong. At that point, Alice decided to give the control to her mother, and that's exactly what both of them wanted. There are many ways to gain control over another human being. Guilt is on the top of the list. Let's start by realizing that no one can make you feel guilty. *Only you can decide whether or not you're guilty.*

Undoubtedly you get a little hot under the collar if someone accuses you of something you're not guilty of. And if you are guilty, a mature person will try to rectify the situation. Guilt is a senseless emotion to begin with. You can only be guilty for something you did that if given the chance to do again, you would do differently. Lock it in your memory bank not to ever repeat the same action again and if it can't be corrected this time, learn from it. Absolutely nothing can be gained from agonizing about it.

But back to Alice. She tried to explain to her mother why she wanted to do the eulogy. And the more she tried, the more she gave her own self-control to her mother.

No amount of food made Alice feel better (as I'm sure you're not surprised to hear). Obviously it didn't help her win back any of the control she had given her mother. Anyway, at that point, I made what sounded like a silly suggestion. "I think it would be a wonderful idea if you were to sit down and write your mother *her* eulogy."

"But Barbara, my mother is still living," Alice replied.

"But", I told her, "so much the better. If you do it now, you could send it to her for her approval. That way she can edit it and add anything you may have forgotten. She'll make sure you don't omit the fact that you were sent to summer camp every year, and that you had tennis and pottery lessons, and a whole multitude of other things you have forgotten to be thankful for. This way you could *give* your mother complete control and you wouldn't have to *lose* control. You could just give it away—and that seems to be what both of you wanted in the first place." In short, we ended up with a very touched mother, and one very delighted, relieved—and thinning—daughter.

That story may sound ludicrous to you, but it was very real to Alice. She is learning how to hold on to and dole out control in the methods and allotments *she* approves of, including her weight. If you have allowed yourself to use your lack of control as an excuse to gain or maintain excess weight, then you will simply have to become more aware of this power you have over yourself. If you don't, you will never change your life or your eating habits and that sounds like a fairly dire future to me.

Carpe Diem

In the golden days of Rome they had a wonderful saying, as any ex-Latin student can tell you. "Carpe diem," or "seize the day" resounded again and again. That not only means live every day as if it were your last (you've already been doing that), but more precisely, make the most of it, make *this* day the one wherein you learn about control.

Remember, it's the power to direct and regulate. Say this aloud:

I will not tolerate the fat on my body any longer!

And again, this time say it with feeling and meaning. And again. Simply wanting to lose weight won't do it. It never has before. You wanted to lose weight yesterday, but you didn't do anything about it. It is not tolerating fat that will make it melt away. Nothing can exist in your life without your tolerance.

I've been using the words "tolerate" and "tolerance" a lot and I want to take a moment to point out to you the connection between tolerance and control. *Tolerance can be a way of letting other people control you by allowing them to do things you wish they wouldn't.*

Have you ever noticed the difference between fat people and skinny people in their capacity for tolerance? Fat people tolerate just about everything. Know why? Because people look at fatties and assume that they are weak—so they push them around. And you stand for it.

Do any of the following situations apply to you?

- You tolerate the way your friends sometimes treat you because you're afraid that if you speak up and tell them how you feel they may dump you.
- You tolerate the way you look—no makeup, unkempt clothes, bitten fingernails or scuffed shoes—because you feel no one pays attention to you anyway.
- You know that you're really much smarter than your boss, but you feel it's worthless to try to prove it to anyone.
- Maybe worst of all: Your children see you have little control and so they don't respect you.

I bet one or more of those examples sounds all too familiar and that you can add others. And it gives you a shameful feeling right in the pit of your stomach, I know. Because somewhere way down under all that poundage, you and I know that you're a true blue friend, a beautiful person, a steady employee and a caring parent.

But you tolerate what others think about you, even if it's not true. And you can't blame them—because each and every day, you're tolerating your own fat body.

Thin people tend to have a better grip on things and tend not to let things slide. You don't see many corporation executives looking like a blimp. These people are in *control*. In control of their jobs, their diets, themselves.

You know by this time as well as I do that hunger is not the motivating factor to your eating. In fact, your weight problem is the result of a lack of motivation, a refusal to control your eating habits.

Now that you have decided to control your meals, start planning what you will eat for your three meals today. Don't keep telling yourself all the things that you *can't* eat if you want to drop those pounds; tell yourself all the wonderful things you *can* eat. Dwell on the positive results. You can learn to eat three good meals a day instead of fantasizing from meal to meal.

Since you're in control again, you'll start to feel relaxed and relieved. Lots of binging guilt has just dropped its hefty poundage off your shoulders. Uncontrolled eating makes you tense and after you have swallowed fattening food, remorse and depression are not far behind. From now on you are going to say before you eat, "I'm in control of this body, I own it and respect it. I don't need this excess food and I don't want it." Every time you make that decision, you will be stronger. Strength builds strength and weakness builds weakness as sure as night follows day.

Throughout your life, there will always be a power struggle for your control. The very mate who has nagged you about your weight could now suddenly start offering you fattening food. They don't like to lose power, either—and they often feel they're losing their power over you. Likewise, an insecure spouse may fear that a new figure may mean new romance for a formerly fat partner. Wolves in sheep's clothing? Of course not—just people who are used to the hold they have over their world and don't want to let go. And it's an established fact that people who hold themselves in low esteem are much easier to control because they feel so inferior to begin with.

Now that you've decided to take the helm, not only in your eating habits, but in your life in general, you'll be in your family and friends' direct line of fire. People will be upset that they can no longer control your thoughts and actions. They'll say that you've changed since you lost weight, that you're not your same old self. Damn straight! What they really mean is that you're happy, proud and on top of things. They're afraid that the change in you may affect their lives. But you can't be put down any longer, you're treating yourself well for the first time in years—and you should expect others to treat you the same. You no longer have to sell your soul to be liked and accepted. You're alive and well and *in control*...

4

The Truth about Fat

Before we go any further, I think it would be a good idea to see if you can separate fact from fiction when it comes to fat.

Most of us were (I suppose purposely) raised on old wives' tales about food. Of course, nobody knows how these stories got started, but all too often we take them as Gospel truth—especially when it's convenient. Our lovely little grandmother who told us these stories would never lie! Stretch the truth a bit, maybe, but never lie. Mine told me these:

Italians eat spaghetti for dinner every night.
The Irish invented the potato.

Chicken soup made by a Jewish mother will cure anything.

Guess Again!

Want to see how many old wives' tales you fell for? Answer true or false.

There is a cure for obesity.

False. Not that you can't get thin, but cure isn't the right word. One thinks of cure as meaning to get rid of once and for all. Unfortunately, obesity is a condition and a choice—it can be controlled—or be out of control. Curing obesity is like curing alcoholism rather than curing measles. It can reoccur at any moment if you give it a chance.

Overweight people are happier and healthier.

False. Fat and jolly. Great dancers—really light on their feet. I wonder what slim person thought up that one. Everyone wants to look slim and trim and certainly many suffer deep periods of depression while carrying around excess poundage. At Slim-U we find there is an alarming amount of self-hatred that has to be dealt with and resolved before weight loss can be achieved. As we've said many times in this book, much of the obesity in this world is the direct result of low self-esteem.

Overweight people have a glandular problem.

False. I often had a beautiful dream that doctors would discover one day that my fat was being caused by underactive glands and not an overactive mouth. No such luck. The percentage of people with a weight problem caused by malfunctioning glands is very small. About five out of ten people use this excuse and many times succeed in convincing themselves that it's a fact. The easiest way to check on sluggish glands—without worrying about big doctors' bills—is to not eat anything fattening for one week and see how quickly those glands start to work. And then see how quickly the pounds go.

Exercise will just make you eat more.

False. I think I invented this tale so I wouldn't have to move any more than was necessary. Until about ten years ago, sweat was a dirty word to me. But exercise is a release for pent-up tension and anxiety, as well as a method of using up calories and keeping a body fit. Moderate exercise is a regulator for the body's weight. It does not increase the appetite. You can do little things you don't normally do. For example: park the car a little farther away from the mall and walk to the entrance. If that sounds stupid to you, notice this next time you go to a mall. The fatties will waste a tank of gas riding around and around looking for a parking space right next to the front door. If it were possible, they'd park in the store window. If you see a space far from the maddening crowd, take it—whether or not you spot another space close up. Taking a short walk every once in a while won't result in your looking like Bo Derek, but you'll have less of a chance of looking like Brünnhilde.

As you get older, you automatically get fatter.

False. Here's an old wives' tale that sounds as though it were actually manufactured by old wives. But it seems to make sense—you glance around and see so many overweight senior citizens. But here in Ft. Lauderdale, where many people choose to retire and remain very active in the year-round good weather, I see lots of slim, good-looking silver-haired foxes of both sexes. These folks seem to have found the secret of life; staying active and enjoying every day. I hope I'll be fortunate enough to see my sixties, seventies, eighties, and—Lord willing—my nineties, still leaving my fat behind.

Food eaten just before bedtime will burn off faster.

False. I know you can't sleep unless you have cookies and milk before you turn in for the night. Mommie always gave you a snack before bed. She probably would have given you the moon just to get you tucked in for the night. This nighttime snack business is a bad habit that should have been broken long ago. Food eaten just before retiring is actually burned off more slowly because it is activity that helps eliminate the calories and the fat they build. If you have spent an active, productive, happy day, you'll sleep just fine without the midnight attack on the refrigerator.

If you eat faster, you will fill up quicker.

False. Watch people eating in a restaurant. The overweight diners look as if they haven't eaten in a month (and we all know they had three meals before they left the house). They should work for Electrolux, they vacuum the food off their plates so well. There seems to be almost an urgency about the way they consume their food. When large amounts of food are forced into the stomach at a great rate of speed, there is no awareness of the amount going in. It will take the stomach about 20 minutes to signal the brain that it's had enough. Hell, in 20 minutes I used to eat everything in the house but the drapes. Lots of dieters will remain true to their diet all day long and then decide to have "a little something" to reward themselves. From that moment on, all hell breaks loose. Something snaps and we're at it again—anything that isn't bolted to the floor is in danger of being consumed by— The Binger. And twenty minutes may not sound like such a long time right now, but imagine what a pair of fast hands can shove into your mouth in that amount of time.

Everyone who loses weight will regain it.

False. You need never to regain your weight again. But, you've got to change a few things to prevent this from happening. The first and most important thing to remember is that it could happen to you again. That fat is never really lost, you see. It's kept in a safe deposit box at the Fat National Bank at Fat Knox, and it's being held in reserve under your name—you can get it back any time. Forget all your old ideas about obesity. *You* caused it and *you* must be in control of your eating habits now and forever. You must believe that you have the ability to shed the pounds and keep them off. Most importantly—change your attitude about *you*. You deserve to be slim!

It's better to lose weight rapidly—by whatever means possible.

False. The fastest way I know is with a butcher knife. Just slice it off. Now *that's* fast. But I warn you, it smarts. There are as many crazy ways to lose weight quickly as there are crazy people to invent them and/or try them. Just the thing for a world infatuated with instant gratification. Any product or diet group that guarantees you'll lose ten pounds in a week is to be feared. A good rate of weight loss is considered to be five to eight pounds a month. Quickly lost, quickly gained. Dieting should produce two things: it should make you healthier and make you look great. There is no point in losing weight and destroying the body. You'll end up looking like something from *Night of the Living Dead.*

If you lose weight quickly, your stomach shrinks.

False. If it were true that the stomach shrinks and stretches according to the amount of food you eat, can you imagine what my stomach looked like at 211 pounds? At least the size of a Volkswagen. There was no limit to the amount of food I would consume in any given day. If there was one box of cookies, I ate one. If there were two, I ate two. My stomach was so full I felt sick, but I kept on eating. What we think of as a shrinking stomach is just that our appetite becomes adjusted to less quantity.

Skip as many meals as possible to lose weight.

False. Overweight people never skip a meal—they just postpone it until later when there is something they really want to eat. Then they'll say "The only reason I'm eating this is because I didn't have any lunch." A balanced eating program is essential to losing weight. Slim folks get hungry after several hours, but overweight people are *starving* ten minutes after they've eaten.

Diet pills and other gimmicks are faster and better.

False. Diet pills, protein drinks, shots, diet cookies, are like a pair of crutches. They'll help as long as the crutches are reinforcing, but take the crutches away and the person will fall. All the gimmicks to lose weight are just that—gimmicks. You can't live on them forever and when you stop, the weight will return at an alarming rate of speed.

Eat grapefruit before meals and you will lose more weight.

False. Ha! If that were true, there wouldn't be a fat person in the state of Florida and we'd all be in the commodities market trading in our pork bellies. Stealing a grapefruit would become a Federal offense and all the culprits would be easy to find—very skinny people with pimples all over their faces from too much citric acid. Don't get me wrong—grapefruit contains vitamin C and that's good for you, so go ahead and eat them. But don't expect any miracles.

If you quit smoking you will gain weight.

False. Smoking doesn't have anything to do with getting fat, nor does the fact that you have quit have anything to do with your gaining. You may find you don't know what to do with your hands, but a resourceful person can find something worthwhile without too much trouble. I hope that by getting this far into the book you have conditioned your brain to realize that fat is caused by *eating*. Slim people all over the world have quit smoking and have maintained their weight. Isn't it interesting that no matter how often slim people go on vacations, attend parties, have crises or quit smoking, they manage to stay slim? If smoking keeps people slim, why are there so many fat smokers?

Losing weight will make you weak and tired.

False. If that were a true statement, then overweight people would have more energy than God. If you're silly enough to try crash dieting, then and only then will losing weight drain you and your energies. That's because you are not eating properly, not because your body's getting lighter.

All foods marked "dietetic" are much lower in calories.

False. And may I add, "Beware!" Many of these products are reduced in caloric count, but not necessarily all of them. *Dietetic* simply means there is no sugar added, making the product acceptable for people with diabetes. The frightening part about obese people seeing that word on a package is that they automatically assume they can eat twice as much. There simply are not that many diet foods. What is a diet chicken? Where do you buy a diet apple or orange? It's all just food, and I hope I'm not disappointing you by telling you that *everything* contains calories. There is no food known to God or man that is totally without calories.

The food allowed on a diet contains no calories.

False. Hey, can't you read? As I explained in the last answer, all food contains calories. People often think that all foods eaten on a diet will be unpleasant because they contain no calories. But what is actually done on any healthy, sensible diet plan is that foods are selected from each food group with the least amount of calories, plus foods that will specifically help burn the calories already accumulated in the body.

If my mother is obese, I will automatically be overweight.

False. In this case, heredity is not the main factor, which should be a comforting fact to most parents as offspring tend to blame all our other problems and shortcomings on the old folks at home. The reason we often see more than one overweight person in a house is simple. They tend to eat the same foods—usually fattening. If one member of the family is not overweight, they'll say she is a poor eater. Fat mothers need an eating buddy and the kids are so available.

A fat baby is much healthier than a thin baby.

False. Grandma might think so, but your doctor will tell you differently. Overweight children walk later, talk later, and so on. If you've never had a loving uncle grab one fat little cheek in each hand and pinch while saying "Now look at the cheeks on this kid," you've never known pain. My daughter's pediatrician always said "Keep them slim. They've got the whole world to grow in."

If you are overweight as a child, you will always be overweight.

False. However, be warned: because a fat child has developed more fat cells than a slim child, they will have to fight harder to keep those fat cells empty. Much of the time, as grown-ups, when we see that some of our friends can eat more than we can and not gain, it's for that very reason. Those fat cells are still there, waiting to be filled up. So let's empty those cells, gang!

Overweight children are a sign of prosperity.

False. Nothing could be less true. It's an indication that either mom doesn't understand that good eating habits are important (or, worse yet, doesn't even know what they are), or that too many of the wrong foods are available to the child. In today's world of fast food chains, many kids think that the only meal that doesn't come out of a white bag with pictures on it is Thanksgiving dinner. The average quicky hamburger contains about 1,000 calories.

The easiest way to get an overweight person to lose weight is by shaming them into it.

False. Shame. Terrific word, isn't it? It should be struck from every dictionary on the face of the earth. It seems to be one of the first words a child hears— "Shame on you" for almost everything. And the sad part is, it doesn't work. It does nothing but produce guilt, and we've all had experience with what the direct result of guilt is—eating ourselves into a coma. The best thing to do is make the correct foods available, encourage less eating, and give praise for *any* weight loss, no matter how small. Try to remember that no one wants to be fat, including us. Substitute love for shame. It produces much better results.

If you get sick, it's better to have some fat to fall back on.

False. Take a walk through any hospital and count the number of overweight patients. Ask what their ailment is and I'll bet my new suede boots that it's connected to their obesity. I saw a bumper sticker a few years back that read "God loves fat people." If that's true, I wonder why He gives us more heart attacks, strokes and high blood pressure problems.

Alcohol is not fattening because it burns right off your body.

False. Don't believe it for a minute. It may burn off when you're using it in cooking, but if it burned right off when we drank it, we wouldn't get drunk. First of all, alcohol has no nutritive value, but is a highly concentrated type of food with an extremely high caloric count. Let's face it—it's bad enough to be fat, and it's bad enough to be an alcoholic, but a fat alcoholic? Whew!

Now you can leave your fat behind forever.

True! True, true at last! No more squishy tushie, no more plump rump. Horray!

How'd you do expelling all those old wives' tales. I know you love to keep score, so here we go. If you got them all right, then you never should have had a weight problem. Half right, you should have no trouble taking it off. And as for you folks who got them all wrong, you had better get busy before you explode!

How to Stop Lying to Yourself

We've just been through all these old wives' tales and found that every last one of them was full of baloney. Some of them may have seemed ridiculous to you, but I assure you, there are people who believe every last one of them—lots of people. And I'll bet you fell for a couple of them. Lord knows there were lots of years I took many of them for the Gospel truth. Now I ask myself why. Some of those stories don't make a bit of sense.

Ever have a friend or relative die and find yourself refusing to believe that it's really true? Or talk yourself into believing that something is going to work out that is clearly irreversible? I think we all have. It's a mode of protection we often use when our mind is not ready to accept the inevitable, whether it be death, taxes or obesity. The problem is, many people never give up their fantasies. They keep believing that everything will straighten out with time. Well, Uncle Chester isn't going to come back, the tax money you need is not going to fall out of the sky and none of those old wives' tales is going to come true. Stop lying to yourself!

When I said being fat is a choice, some of you probably thought it a strange thing to say. After all, one doesn't sit down and say "I think I'll be fat." What I'm getting at here is that we tend to lie to ourselves. We really *have* made a choice to be fat, no matter how unconsciously we've done it. In fact, the more unconscious a decision we make, the harder it's going to be to open our own eyes. Then we start to lie to ourselves pretending that we haven't noticed that we've gained another ten pounds, and another. We know we're lying, too, when we say we'll start our diet tomorrow. Why lie to such a swell person?

Well, there is a reason we lie to ourselves. We're the ones we must report to, we know all our own bad secrets, we know how we're cheating and defeating ourselves every time we pop another cookie into that bottomless gorge until we come to that final decision to take control of our lives and believe that we can control our weight. Making that decision and admitting to yourself that you've been lying to the most important person in your life is the hardest part of all. You should be delighted to hear that. It's all a lot easier from there on in.

Here's something I do when I find I'm doing things behind my own back. When I realize that I've eaten something I shouldn't or overlooked a task that really needed doing, I write it down. Now I'm not into public humiliation. I hide these little slips of paper, I don't throw myself at the mercy of my family by posting it on the refrigerator. There's nothing wrong with doing it that way either if you really think you need occasional pep talks from the family. But I find that just putting pen to paper and admitting my dishonesty to myself gives me a great sense of relief and a reminder that I'm still pulling cheating tricks behind everyone's back—especially my own!

Whether you're fooling yourself, or you're believing an old wives' tale, you're *choosing to believe what suits you.* The frightening thing is that once you start doing this, it becomes easier and easier to tell yourself little white lies. Soon enough, they'll be giant whoppers. Do you ever cringe when someone asks "What happened to that cake I just brought home?" Do you not only cringe, but say you never saw it when you just polished it off? I sure have, and I'll tell you, it made me feel awful (the cake *and* the lying). One lie leads to another and soon you're lying about things other than food and the next thing you know you don't even believe yourself anymore. Then who do you turn to when you need help?

Sit down right now and go through the old wives' tales again. Go through all the ones you answered as false. You may have marked them as false while taking this test alone, knowing the answers in your heart of hearts. But have you ever told yourself in a convenient situation that those questions were true? When you wanted a little "dietetic" candy? Or wanted to think your fat little two-year-old niece was really in the pink? Try to think of three things you've done recently that you've managed to make yourself think were allowable. Just write them down on a piece of paper. Now look at them. Feel better? Kind of like going to confession, but you don't have to worry about the ten Our Fathers—you just have to try not to do it again. Finally, tear up the paper into little, tiny pieces and flush them down the toilet. You know where the answers really are...

5

44D Is the Loneliest Number

There really isn't much that's worse in the loneliness category—except maybe Christmas with Scrooge—than being fat. And half the reason is because no one could get near you even if they tried. No one takes you to the movies because they would have to pay for three seats. No one wants to take you out to dinner because it's too expensive. And no one takes you to an amusement park because you can't even fit in the Dodge 'ems. So you sit home with the nice presents they give you instead—popcorn poppers, a subscription to *Gourmet,* a giant box of Bill Blass designer chocolates. Sounds pretty grim, right? Maybe it even sounds a little like your life. So what's keeping you from changing it?

Is It Failure You Fear?

Fail is certainly a four letter word, and one we fatties have used regularly over our fat years. In the past, we've accepted failure like a speeding ticket—we know we've done something wrong and we take the consequences resignedly. Failure to lose weight has made us feel much worse than before we had started whatever diet it was this time around. Once again we've proved to ourselves that we're not only fat, but we just can't do anything about it. We tell ourselves we have no control, and the whole thing is useless. The self-esteemometer starts to plummet.

Well, we were right about one thing—we had no control. Most diets take the control from you the minute you start. From day one your life is regulated to mid-morning snacks of three grapefruit sections and one lettuce leaf, tea with a cracker at 4:07 P.M., two ounces of club soda upon retiring, etc., etc. You start a diet like this and think "Great! All I have to do is follow orders and I will be beautiful in two short weeks." Ha! My fat behind you will be. First of all, _no one_ likes to be ordered around like that. After a while, mutiny is bound to occur, if only for the sake of showing the author of the latest diet book that you know who's really boss. Just tell someone they've got to do what you say, and they'll take a 180° turn. In the fat world, of course, this is known as binging. So there goes the West Point style of losing weight.

Now I'm not saying you can't lose weight on any of those diets—obviously you can. But when the regimentation is over, who do they put back into the pilot's seat? You. You're supposed to be in control again, now, and you're lost.

Now you'll fail because you were never in control in the first place!

Sure, we give good guidelines and advice at Slim-U, and lots of healthy recipes such as the ones in the back of this book. But from week to week, weigh-in to weigh-in and every minute in between, *you* are the one who chooses whether or not to be in control. *You* are what makes a diet work, not dry toast. As far as fat and diets are concerned, "Nothing ventured, nothing gained" does not hold true. Do not, I repeat, do not make it your motto.

If we feared failure in everything we did, nothing would ever get accomplished. You have to look at losing weight as a daily battle—the only battle you win when you lose. I'll find that some of my Slim-U members won't show up for a meeting because they know they've gained a pound or two, and they're ashamed to come in and admit it. (Hell, anyone who says they never cheat is a liar. Except for me, of course.) So then I have to give this person a call and assure him or her that all is not lost (by a long shot) and they've just got to try harder the next week. There are some people who *want* to fail, just to tell themselves they've blown it again and get back to the serious business of eating—or should I say overeating.

Just remember that you haven't failed until you've stopped trying. Don't accept failure—it's easy to jump in the proverbial sack with it, because guilt, remorse and low self-esteem are comfortable and familiar bedfellows. But think about this: did you ever think that maybe what you really feared was success?

I know that sounds stupid, but listen to this. I had the manuscript for this book for a long time before I ever *dared* to submit it to a publisher. I talked about it to a friend one day who was egging me on to try to get it published. "Well why not, B.Z.?" he was saying to me, "what have you possibly got to lose?" I told him I didn't have anything at all to lose, but that I was just afraid that no one would buy it and I'd fail. Well, he didn't go along with that. "You're not afraid of failing," he insisted. "You're afraid of success." Naturally I told him he was off his rocker. Who, after all, would be afraid of having a bestselling book? Who'd be afraid of being recognized on the streets? Who'd be afraid of appearing on talk shows, or touring around the country helping other people like myself lose weight?

I was beginning to see what he meant.

The responsibilities of success can be overwhelming. When you've been overweight for any length of time, the new light in which you'll be seen as a slim person is frightening. It can be scary to have to politely turn down married men, or take on the new pressures of a promotion to a very visible position you never would have gotten as a fat employee. But I'll let you in on a secret. In the long run, it's a lot easier than looking at yourself in the mirror every morning and seeing what you saw this very day. Fail is a four-letter word. Success isn't.

Mapping Out New Strategies

Are you all beginning to think I'm a real bitch because I refuse to lead you around by the nose (or spare tire) and tell you what to do every minute? Well, I can help you map out some new strategies just to get you going in the right direction. You can have all the good intentions in the world, but can continue to go around in circles for quite a while. A little shove doesn't hurt. Especially a little shove toward motivation and away from procrastination.

Motivation is a beautiful concept. It absolutely leads straight to success. All the calorie counting in the world won't help you lose an ounce if you're not sincerely committed to taking off weight. And to do that, you've got to be motivated. Many psychologists will tell you that your motivation to diet may be the single most important factor determining the success or failure of your efforts to become slimmer.

To find out just how motivated you are, make a list of five reasons why you want to lose weight. Don't read any further—just jot down some of your thoughts on a slip of paper and put them aside for the moment. If you can't come up with five reasons, this may explain the difficulties you have in trying to take off those extra pounds. In short, maybe you just don't think enough of yourself at this point in your life to want to do something about the way you look. It's important to your diet to establish your motivation before you dive in—then you know what you're striving for, and why. Here are some dieting motivations I have gathered to help you get started if you're having trouble coming up with some yourself.

I must lose weight because:

1. Clothes don't look good on me at my present weight, and my weight and my physical appearance are important aspects of the impression I make on people in my life and the people I'm about to meet.
2. I feel uncomfortable, sluggish and "dumpy" when I am overweight.
3. I wish to become more attractive to my husband, wife, boyfriend, girlfriend, etc. and be attractive to the people I meet.
4. I feel my weight is not appropriate to my body size and that it's unhealthy for me to be carrying around this extra baggage.
5. I am embarrassed that others can see by looking at me that my eating is out of control—and then they know that *I* must be out of control.
6. I feel that my weight detracts from my physical appearance to the extent that it might be holding me back on my job.
7. I don't like to engage in activities which require that I wear revealing clothing. It shows how overweight I am and this limits my experiences.
8. My weight makes me reluctant to meet new people and this holds me back socially.

9. I feel that my weight problem might make my relatives, children, spouse or friends ashamed of me.
10. I know that I feel more attractive, happier and more comfortable when I weigh less.

Any of these motivations match yours? Probably a couple of them come pretty close. Not all of those I have listed here are specifically mine, but they are all reasons I've heard dieters give at one time or another for why they want to be thinner. Actually, anyone who is overweight can probably relate to most of them, if not all.

It's good to stop worrying every once in a while about The Diet and sit down and remember exactly why you don't want to be fat. It puts your wishes and your goal in perspective.

So, now that we've come up with the reasons why we want to lose weight, let's make sure that we don't blow it by procrastinating. All the theorizing at Harvard won't help you lose an ounce—if you lose weight, it's because you've done something about it. Again, we're afraid we won't succeed, so we tell ourselves that we can lose weight anytime we want to—we just don't want to right now. In this way, we don't have to admit to ourselves that we're not going to do it at all. Being a doer requires three things that aren't so easy to come by: effort, to stay away from illegal food; risk of going out and being constantly tempted; and change, which is difficult to accept, especially when it must be self-imposed as in dieting. It's always easier to talk about how someone else has performed than to be a performer.

Look at these two typical instances of procrastinating behavior. One is not tackling addictions, the old I'll-quit-when-I'm-ready technique. As I said a moment ago, we put it off because deep down we really don't believe we can do anything about it. Another instance is to claim you're going to go on a diet, but say you're going to start on Monday, or after Christmas (commonly used during July). Somehow these days never arrive, and the ones when you have to go to the dentist do. Odd, isn't it?

Let's check out some techniques, then, for getting rid of procrastinating behavior.

Make a decision to live five minutes at a time.

Don't think of tasks in long-range terms. To think of how long you have to be on a diet is instant death for that diet. Think about now and try to use up a five-minute period doing what you want, and refuse to put off anything that will bring you satisfaction.

Begin your diet this moment.

There's absolutely no reason that's good enough to postpone your diet any longer. Put this book down for a second and do one push-up as your beginning exercise project. That's how you tackle problems. With action. *Now, do it!* The only thing holding you back is you.

Look hard at your life.

Are you doing what you would choose to be doing if you knew you had six months to live? Our total lifetime is a mere speck. It just doesn't make sense to delay anything.

Eliminate useless words from your vocabulary.

No, not those words. They're very useful. But words like "hope," "wish" and "maybe" aren't. They are tools of procrastination. Be aware of these words creeping into sentences and rout them out.

If you want things to change, don't complain, do something about them. Be a doer, not a wisher, hoper or critic. Don't think if you wait around things will get better. They may change, but they won't get better. Your life only gets better because you've done something constructive to make it so. Take things into your own hands and avoid typical procrastinating behavior like the following:

Staying in a job you hate.
Hanging onto a relationship that has gone sour.
Not tackling social diseases such as obesity, alcoholism, smoking, drugs.
Putting off menial tasks: cleaning, ironing, sewing, etc.
Avoiding a confrontation with others.
Being afraid to move to another city, state, etc.
Using the line "I'm busy."
Using tiredness to put things off.
Getting suddenly sick when faced with an unpleasant task.
"I just don't have the time to do it."
Constantly looking toward the future instead of enjoying the present.
Refusing to get a physical check-up.
Being bored.
Living your entire life for your children or spouse.
Deciding to start your diet tomorrow.

Procrastination allows you to escape—you never have to change, you can just plug away every day at being your dreary old self. How exciting. You can go on blaming others for your unhappy state and live in a dream world. So, right now, avoid procrastination and try this: start something right now that you've been putting off (a diet is a good idea if nothing else comes to mind); set a designated time to do something you want accomplished. I can't tell you how good doing these little things will make you feel, but if you take my advice *right now*, you'll know yourself in a matter of minutes.

Slim vs. Fat: Pros and Cons

At this point I thought it might be helpful to make a chart so we can clearly see the pros and cons of being slim as opposed to being fat. Observe:

The Slim World
>   Pros
>   Lots of attention and sexual passes
>   Feeling like Chris Evert-Lloyd/John McEnroe
>   Looking like Lauren Hutton/Christopher Reeve
>   Liking what I see in the mirror
>   Confidence to ask for a raise—and getting it!
>   Grocery bills have been cut in half

>   Cons
>   Have spent so much money on fancy new clothes that I've none left to buy new date book

The Fat World
>   Pros
>   On a first-name basis with every checkout cashier at each grocery store in a five-mile radius

>   Cons
>   My spouse hasn't missed The Late Movie in six years
>   Finding doctor's bills, high blood pressure pills, etc. too high
>   Feel like it's easier for me to roll somewhere rather than walk
>   Have a penchant for bikinis (I can dream, can't I?)
>   Beginning to have a hard time getting through revolving doors
>   Hate myself

I rest my case.

6

Someone Special

Our attitudes about ourselves are constantly changing. Being overweight causes our attitude about ourselves to flip-flop—and in our case, mostly flop. Because each time we get on the scales and see we've gained a pound or two, we lose a point of self-esteem. This happens to slim people, too, because they tend to realize better than obese people that they're losing control. They are more aware of it and their alarm goes off a lot sooner. But basically, from day to day, our attractiveness to ourselves can go up and down like the Dow Jones.

A question I often ask my Slim-U members can have as many different answers as there are days, but overall, it gives a fair impression of what an individual thinks about oneself—and often how he or she *pigeonholes* oneself. It's a question that always seems to shock everyone when they're asked, but one which people seem to have an almost immediate answer to in each instance. I'd like to introduce you to someone special in this chapter, and I'll start off by asking that very question.

Finding Out Who

If you were to give yourself a title, what would it be?

What was the first thing that came to your mind? Joe's Wife? Ellen's Mother? Lauren's Daughter? Paul's Boss, Mike's Friend—Fatso, maybe? Of course we can give ourselves several titles, all of which may be important to us. But did you find when you answered that question, the first answer you came up with was an other-related title? By that I mean a title dependant on someone else's relationship to you, as in those titles above. Or worse yet did you settle for big, fat blob.

There are other titles that are inner-directed and could make you feel terrific were you to concentrate on giving yourself one. Try some of these on for size (none of them are 22½'s)—Fun Queen of the Greater Northeast, Smartest Account Executive in My Office, Most Compassionate Person I Know, even (shudder) Best Cook in Town. I love being Bill's Wife, Bilinda's Mother, Susan's Boss and friend to my Slim-U members; but most importantly the title I love most, find the most pride in and fight the hardest to maintain is "Barbara Zara, Important Person." Best of all, I didn't make up this title—it's true.

What would you like to be that you aren't now?

I know, I know, *slim*. But in a long-range sense, that's not likely to be your first answer. And it's not a silly question. The silly part is, why aren't you headed in that direction now? As a for instance: there was this tall, homely guy (albeit skinny) with hardly any education, not much of a conversationalist, who thought he might be able to become President of the United States. Poor, crazy Abe Lincoln, he really didn't stand a chance. Lindbergh said he'd fly across the Atlantic Ocean! And joke of all bad jokes—a *Polish* Pope?! You want to hear the best one? I though I could write a book—even funnier than that, I thought you might read it. In short—

GET OFF YOUR ASS!

All you have to do is get going *now* to change your attitude about yourself and what you can accomplish.

What's your definition of being happy?

Usually, what's uppermost in your mind pops out as an answer first: more money, a new car, being slim, a divorce. But you know as well as I do that when you sit down and think about it, the answer goes much deeper than that. It's more likely to be peace of mind, loving and being loved, starting a task, completing it, and knowing in your heart you've done your best. Perhaps a better tennis game might be next on the list, but how about staying cool in the summer and warm in the winter, having someone to come home to, a good night's sleep and the strength to greet the morning with excitement. All in all, aren't we each happiest when we know we're doing our best?

Do you believe someone can be truly happy?

Believe it! You're probably happier at this moment than you realize. Love, fun, happiness are things you seldom take stock of until you've lost them. It's kind of like when you sprain a finger—you have no idea how much you use it until it's out of commission. And then when it heals, you go back to taking your good health—both physical and mental—for granted again. Try not to look back to what was or forward to what might be your happiest moment—it could very well be *now*, so appreciate it!

Do you depend on others to make you happy?

We're sort of back at the question of what your title would be. If you're depending on someone else for your own happiness, you're in for or may be experiencing some rough times. I've got news for you. It isn't the main function of every other human being to see to your happiness. So many marriages fail because we feel it is our spouse's *duty* to make us happy, and when they become involved in the every day world of simply trying to keep their (not your) head above water, we end up feeling betrayed. Some women, for example, attempt to find all their happiness through their children when they're small and when the kids grow up and take off, they're resentful. The kids have deserted them, and so has their happiness. In reality, finding your own happiness is like a job; you work with people, form a team where everyone tries to help each other out, and you make friends and maybe some enemies. The important part is that you're at the center of the circle, reaching out for two-way dialogue. Just remember—*you're at the center, and it all comes back to you*. So *you* are the one that makes it work—you're the one that makes you happy.

Is happiness a choice?

Absolutely. Everyone knows a sourpuss or a real curmudgeon who is miserable all the time just because they feel like being feisty. Truth is, they may be loving every minute of it. Or if they're not, they're just not opening themselves up enough to receive any love. There can be a real fear of happiness if one thinks he'll lose control, just as there is that fear of success. But basically, you choose to be happy by enjoying everything to its fullest—at my age, I think the pleasure of opening my eyes each morning is a miracle! Even a cup of tea, clean sheets, a kiss, hug, a birthday card or a surprise phone call from someone we miss are things we take for granted. Yet if we *didn't* have things like this, I'll bet you we'd feel somewhat empty and unhappy. Boy, those things add up.

Can you learn to be happy?

Your figure shows that you've done a damn good job of learning to be unhappy, so the converse is probably true. Through guilt and a number of other things, you manage to teach yourself to be unhappy and you're carrying it around in the form of fat. Children, for example, don't realize when they're "supposed to" be happy or unhappy. It's we grown-ups who teach them to become more serious and shoulder them with the responsibilities and wishes that are our own. *If we can learn to live our own lives, and not someone else's, we can be as happy as we wish.* As they say, "There is no way to happiness, happiness is the way."

Do you look for others to blame for your unhappiness?

For example, do you blame others for your being over-weight? "My parents always insisted I clean my plate," "I feel I should eat what my kids left," "I always felt so out of it because my brother was so much better looking than I," etc., etc. It always seems so *true* when we're dealing with our own lives. But think about it...if you've ever been associated with someone who always places the blame on someone else (and in many cases it might be *you),* their stories always have a bit less than the ring of truth to them. In the end, you often find you'd rather not be in their tiresome company at all. Don't get me wrong, we all do it. But next time you hear yourself say "I never get the breaks"..."all my luck is bad" ..."because of him I missed my big chance"..."who *wouldn't* be unhappy with my wife, kids, mother, boss, blah, blah, blah"...next time you hear that coming out of your own mouth, remember that *you're* the only one who can do anything about it, not your semi-captive audience.

Do you love yourself?

You should, and I can give you one irrefutable reason why. You're the only one of your kind—"when they made you, they threw the mold away" my mother always said (in what I chose to hear as a tone of great pride). In your day-to-day living, you probably manage to swing things your way so treat yourself well if you feel you deserve it, and generally try not to let people step all over you—even if it's something so small as cutting ahead of you in a line. Those actions prove that you look out for #1 first—so doesn't that mean you love yourself? Then take it all the way! Celebrate the fact that you—and only you—are you. Share it with yourself and others. And give yourself that special treat of showing yourself how wonderful you are by becoming slim. You deserve it!

Do you find it hard to express your love to others?

I've always had a thought that seems really corny, but I've found that, in the long run, it's helped me treat people better. All of us have wished at one time or another that we could bring back someone who we loved and tell them the things we wished we had said before he or she died. We would have said how much we enjoyed their humor—or simply that we loved them. Maybe it's just a bit morbid, but it's often useful to treat people as if you were never going to see them again. Imagine! It would be like Christmas all year. So next time you realize you haven't hugged your kids, or kissed your mother, or called someone you should have, give it a try. "If I told my husband I loved him, he'd drop dead!"

said a friend of mine when I suggested this tactic. Faint, maybe, but never drop dead.

Are you terribly afraid of rejection?

Although we all love to be stroked and petted, we all know that isn't always available to us, even from our loved ones. Even your lover, husband, son or daughter will use rejection as a way to control you—it's human nature, and really just a more subtle way of arguing. But as long as you know that you've tried your best, there's no need to feel down in the dumps at someone's hotheaded treatment. Holding back one's love just to prove a point is hurting not only the rejectee, but the rejector as well.

How do you react to rejection?

OK, OK, let's face it. *Not everyone in the entire world is going to like you.* Yup, that's right. And not everything you do or say is going to be accepted. That's OK. Everyone's got different ideas of what's best. The important thing is, do *you* like you? If yes, terrific, but why are you overweight? If you aren't completely satisfied with you, it's time you go about changing you, and I guarantee you, losing weight is going to make you feel *terrific*!

Do you dwell on rejection?

Let's not get too philosophical about this, let's just set the stage. You are at a party feeling like a combination of Cleopatra, Mata Hari and Bo Derek. Just as you are about to take out your pen to autograph a few cocktail napkins, some handsome dude strolls over to you (as you ready your pen) and says "Aren't you a friend of my mother's?" Now, tell the truth. If every other person at that entire party comes over and actually drools on your dress, what will you remember about that party? And for how long—a week, a month, forever? But why should you donate any part of your life to someone who makes you feel badly? What have they got, the key to wisdom, the absolute truth from above? Look at it this way, using this highly technical two-point method:

1. It is just their opinion.
2. Who asked them anyway?

Do you live in the present moment, today, this minute?

If you have learned to, you have found the secret to living life to its fullest. "I can't wait till we go on vacation in two weeks," "I wish it were Friday," "Only ten years till I retire." They say anticipation is half the fun—but why wish your life away? The most precious thing about this moment, today, is that it never was before and never will be again. Maybe you're overweight, but aren't there plenty of good things around you that make everything worthwhile? You can remember the past, of course, but that's for purposes of enjoyment. You can plan for the future, but not at the expense of losing today. You're never promised tomorrow, but today, this moment is yours. Enjoy!

Do you feel guilty about yesterday and afraid of tomorrow?

If I could choose to wipe one word out of the dictionary, it would be guilt. Isn't it nice how people want to share it with us, give it to us, heap it up to our necks? When I catch on that I'm chatting with the East Coast Distributor of Guilt, I tell him I'm not interested in buying. He can peddle his wares elsewhere. And if you pay attention to today, how can you be afraid of tomorrow? Hell, I'm too busy with today to worry about tomorrow! Today took care of itself . . . no reason why tomorrow won't.

Do you look for people's faults, or can you accept them for what they are?

People who are quick to point out the faults of others are really saying "That isn't the way *I* would do it, so you must be wrong." Aren't there many ways to do one thing? If you find that you're picking others apart a great deal, maybe it's because you're trying to draw attention *away* from the way you're conducting your own life. It's a funny equation, but when we find we like who and what *we* are, others seem to have fewer faults.

Do you feel loved by the people you love?

If not, you're loving the wrong people. I intend to love Robert Redford forever, but at least I realize that's a fault, because I haven't heard a thing through the Hollywood grapevine about the way he feels about me. Other than that, I think I love the right people, and they return my love. It's just give and take, but the trick is, you've got to do both the giving *and* the taking. There are people you can tell a thousand times a day how much you love them, but they never believe it. If they're down enough to feel they don't deserve to be loved, they just won't accept it. I'll tell you though, believe it or not, and you may think it's silly when you live in Boise, Idaho, *I* love you. I understand what you're going through, and that you're trying to better yourself, and I truly love you for that.

Do you look for your faults? Can you accept yourself as a whole person?

You're going to be whole, with or without your faults. However, you can be a healthy or unhealthy whole, and if one of your faults is obesity, you're sure to be unhealthy. Get out your good intentions and put them to use—look for your faults and make it your business to better yourself. Nothing's written in stone, no matter how old you are, fat you are, dishonest you are. I'll tell you something...you may *think* you're pretty foxy at looking out for #1, but you aren't truly successful at it until you make yourself the best you can be.

Do you realize you are a miracle?

You sure are! The most humbling experience of my life was the first time I held my daughter Bilinda in my arms. I knew the procedure of conception, in what sequence the child's body was formed, and I sure as hell had learned the pain of childbirth. But none of what I had learned about pregnancy and childbirth told me where she *really* came from. Could anyone on earth design something so perfectly—even Armani? To me, she was an absolute miracle, as is the birth of every child. And a miracle doesn't stop being a miracle as it grows older, does it? We have such a short time on earth to appreciate all the miraculous people we encounter... and so little time to appreciate *ourselves*. Being fat is no way to do it, either. So when I say "Live it up!" that does not necessarily mean "Eat a cupcake."

Removing "If" From Your Vocabulary

All these questions have referred to *you*, how *you* feel about yourself, what bothers you about you and the way you lead your life. Basically, what would happen "if" you rid yourself of guilt and feelings of rejection, how it might feel "if" you lived in the present, or what it could feel like "if" you were happy. Well, I personally think "if" is another one of those useless words and, may I add, there is no "'if' I lose this weight." It's *when*. When is *now*. Not that all your excess weight is going to just drop off of you this very moment, but there's no time like the present to start. It's all the "ifs" that lie out there in the future that have caused you to lose control of your life, led you to lead an existence that is less than ideal. Since you deserve the best, you should present yourself with it—no one else is going to, believe me.

These questions made you dig a little deeper, and you either liked doing that or not. If they made you uncomfortable, there's a reason why—you must know you're not giving yourself a fair chance. If you were pleased with the questions—and your answers—then congratulations, you've probably got a good handle on what's happening in your life. Not that there's no room for improvement, mind you. If these probings truly bothered you, start the ball rolling. You can only succeed on your own, but I'm willing to bet that your loved ones are behind you...and after all, that's why I'm here, isn't it? Just remember one thing:

Nothing in your life will change for the better until you decide that change is needed.

I'm afraid the change machine can't be put on automatic pilot. So rev up and take off! And, oh, by the way...
What did you say your title is?

THREE

Where Did It Come From?

7

Truth or Consequences: A Quiz

Ah, wouldn't it be a wonderful world if we were suddenly to discover that our reasons for being overweight were due to a lack of knowledge and understanding about what to eat and what *not* to eat. If you've been fighting fat most of your life, you should be aware that mainlining cookies, ice cream, potato chips, candy, etc. has resulted in you waddling around most of your life, but they sure as hell weren't the cause. The truth is, everyone in the world basically knows what's fattening and what's not—that's why this book is a diet book about people and what makes them tick, and not a diet book about food.

Let's establish another fact. Your hands and mouth aren't the culprits of your obesity, either. Place the blame—

and the credit—where it belongs. Your mind. Nothing transpires until your brain gives the signal.

There is never one definitive answer to why people do things. And yet there is an alarming similarity in the behavior of dieters. We of the Constant Diets have spent years researching foods—what contains the most and least calories, carbohydrate grams, sugar, salt, etc., etc. We've made charts, diagrams and outlines, we've written daily and weekly menus and weighed foods in the kitchens of the world, and when all was said and done, a large percentage of obese people were...obese. Why? Because we've been concentrating on food, and not the reasons we've been overeating. All the fussing and orchestrating has served only one purpose—to convince ourselves that we are truly trying to lose weight when in fact all we are doing is once again removing the responsibility of control from ourselves.

Take a look at the questions I've posed below. Try not to read my comments after each question for a few moments. Instead, give yourself a little time to answer every one truthfully; remember, no one's listening, especially if you aren't talking out loud.

Does your weight affect the way you feel about yourself?

Nothing physical should ever affect the love and respect you have for yourself. Remember, if the world were blind, no one would know if you weighed 97 or 435 pounds. They would be judging you purely on your merits. Well, that's exactly what you should do. Who you are—your beliefs, feelings and actions should be from your heart. Being overweight doesn't make you a lesser person, and more importantly, being slim isn't going to make you a better person. Start by accepting yourself as you are, and love yourself for the good in you. Now, the things you want to change, like your weight, are up to you. It's your choice.

Does being overweight affect the way you live your life?

Yes? I'm not too surprised—it sure affected me. Maybe you said yes because it makes you move a little slower, have a harder time getting into and out of, causes you to be a trifle short of breath. Those answers are universal for fatties like us. But aside from that, how about the deeper truth. Ever hold back from trying something because you're afraid of rejection or failure? Ever wondered if you lost out on a job or a friendship because of your appearance? Well, maybe it was due to your weight problem—and maybe not. But there's only one way to find out. And once you're thin you'll have nothing to blame for failure except you. That's when you get to the real formation of You, an ever-changing and fascinating project. You can't blame fat—you can only realize that it didn't get there all by itself. No guts, no glory.

Do you truly realize that being overweight is a choice?

Hard to acknowledge, I know, but deep down under those layers of fat you keep telling yourself are for hibernation purposes, you are keenly aware that you have a choice. And that's the bad news—you've been making the *wrong* choices. The good news is that every moment is an opportunity to say no to food and make the wiser choices that will make you slim and healthy. Think of it this way—what if obesity was something that just happened to us through no fault of our own. Imagine being stuck with it. Whew! Believe me, I thank someone up there every day that I *had* the choice to be slim. Then I thank myself for opting for that choice.

Do you eat even when you're not hungry?

This is as good a time as any to define hunger. The dictionary says it's "The distress brought about by the lack of food." Well, we've been pretty distressed about the lack of food a few times, gang, but let's face it, the dictionary is talking starvation, not afternoon treats. Ever notice that fatties use the word "starved," not hungry. It sounds much more urgent, and judging from our obesity, we've seen some intensely urgent moments. But I can give an incredibly wise piece of advice that will let you sleep tonight:

You cannot die of hunger between lunch and dinner.

Surprised? Countless experiments have proven this to be a valid statement! And get this—an even more dizzying thought: if we ate when we were *really hungry*, and not for emotional reasons, most days would consist of two small meals.

Do you feel remorseful and guilty because of overeating?

I always did, though I'll say it never helped me lose an ounce. You know, there are only two types of guilt—one when you've done something you wish you hadn't, and one when you haven't done something you wish you had. With overeating, it's usually the first. And oddly enough, we manage to make our mind hold off the guilt until the last crumb of cookie hits our stomach. But oh boy, are we sorry then! Guilt can be used in two ways. You can let it conquer your spirit, and that will keep you from accomplishing the things you want most in life—like being slim. But you can also use guilt as a lesson, to learn enough from it so that you won't do the same thing twice. That's using guilt to your best advantage. Everyone has felt guilty. When you think about it, lifting the weight of guilt from your shoulders is like losing twenty pounds. And just as hard. Try to use it to *your* best advantage.

Do you often binge on fattening foods?

Don't be shy—you're certainly not alone. I've binged so bad I've gotten blisters on my fingers. Binging is a learned habit and a lot of us have studied it closely and earned A + s.

What we've got to remember, though, is that before every binge there's one swift moment of permission giving. You stop, you think, and what do you say to yourself? "This little bit won't hurt me. I'll just enjoy this tiny snack and then go right back on my diet." Well there are two things to be said about that statement. One, there usually isn't an arm that comes out and pins you down after "this little bit." And two, isn't what you're saying more like "I don't give a damn"?

Do you plan ahead for your food orgies?

There are not many questions (except for "Are you having an affair?") that immediately conjure up such a resounding "No!" But we do. We stock up on things we tell ourselves are for the kids or our spouse, and lo and behold, they just happen to be our favorites. Who ever heard of a fat person pigging out on lettuce and fruit?

The worst part of a binge is that it accomplishes absolutely nothing. The orgasmic joy of it lasts about twenty minutes. In that time, we run from the refrigerator to the pantry and back to the refrigerator, eating any combination of food we can get our hands on. The binge will only last twenty minutes, as I indicated, because that's how long it takes for the stomach to notify the brain *"Please,* I've had enough—in fact, I've had more than enough." And, inevitably, when it's over, both your mind *and* your stomach feel awful.

Do you spend a large part of your day thinking about food?

Our first reaction is to say "Are you kidding? I'm too busy to spend my time doing that." Right—shopping, making grocery lists, cooking—all this takes time! Then you buy sweets to "hide for the kids" so they won't spoil their appetites; or do we hide them so no one else knows where they are? Or we'll bake twice as much as we need for that party so we can keep some for you know who. And even if you're not at home all day, there are coffee breaks, endless phone calls for lunch dates, choosing bars for a drink because they have hors d'oeuvres. Getting fat is a full time job!

Do you overeat most when you're alone?

Probably so—I know I always did. We've been taught to feel guilty about eating because we are carrying more than our doctor's prescribed weight. People tend to get after us about it, and even though they do it because they love us, it just makes us crawl into our shell (manicotti or otherwise) more and more. We'll get impatient when waiting for someone to leave or go to bed so we can hit the kitchen. That can sure put a strain on relationships. Or we'll watch for an opportunity to pop something into our mouths, and swallow the food whole for fear of being caught and suffering the embarrassment. There's not one of us who hasn't prayed silently at one time or another for something to slide down our throats before we choked to death in the middle of a cocktail party. Getting caught with a lover was never so painful—or embarrassing! A good rule of thumb is to try not to isolate yourself. Go to bed when your spouse does—chat with someone in the kitchen while you cook, etc.

Do you find sneaking food exciting?

Speaking of an illicit rendezvous! Excitement at doing something you think is wrong is usually a nervous flow of adrenalin that's basically saying "watch out!" And that excitement is soon followed by remorse and guilt. Think back—all the exciting times of sneaking and cheating ice cream sundaes, coffee cakes and peanut brittle made you fat, guilty and depressed in the end. Such excitement we can live without.

After such a binge, do you feel ashamed?

Shame's a pretty strong word, especially if you're on the receiving end. We've all probably used it on someone and I can still remember how bad I felt when my mother said, "I'm ashamed of you." Well, I learned that shame is something people give away that you don't have to take. You can reject it—there's no shame in eating, it is simply a choice. And each choice we make in rejecting our obesity is a step toward self-esteem.

Do you eat sensibly in front of others?

Sure we do. We may eat all day long if we know we're going out to dinner later on with some friends. That's because we know from experience that those who love us most will be the cruelest when they see us stuffing ourselves like a pig. So since we want to be loved and accepted, we attempt to *appear* to be acting as others want us to act. Now that *you've* decided to lose weight, you'll learn to eat sensibly because you want to, not because you're trying to impress someone.

Do you eat compulsively when worried or depressed?

The biggest percentage of our compulsive eating is done in mid-morning. Our next feast starts around three to five in the afternoon, or five to six if you've got a fulltime job. In order to condone our morning raid on the kitchen, we've got to find something to make us nervous. Something like too much housework or noisy kids. Afternoon assaults on food can be justified by the unnerving fact that the older kids are stampeding in from school. Then dinner's got to be made and that alone can put you into a frenzy. Or maybe there was something you didn't get done or your husband didn't kiss you before he left the house, or your mother-in-law called, or

the dog threw up on the carpet (you probably overfed him).
Any of these things could activate the old nervous system.
Ready, set *eat!* If we need a reason to be fat I guess nerves are
good enough.

Then there's our old friend, depression. You don't even
need a recent situation to become depressed. On some days
when you're looking for a license to gorge you may go back to
your childhood in order to dredge up something horrendous
enough to feed you and your depression for several days. A
good week of depression can run into eight or ten pounds.

Compulsive eating is an immediate thing; it must be
done quickly, without thinking. If you stop for a moment and
think of how much obesity has hurt you, you can curb that
compulsion to eat.

Do you always have a ready excuse for being obese?

I think my second book will be entitled *An Encyclopedia
of Excuses for Being Fat.* "If I even *look* at food I gain weight";
"Everything I eat turns into instant fat"; "My whole family is
fat" (this is an excuse?); "It's in my genes!" It's in your jeans
alright. Will my encyclopedia be fact or fiction, you wonder.
Depends on who's reading it. If you truly believe it's fact,
then it will remain fact—always. Only when you see that it's
fiction, written by you, will you be able to rewrite the script.

*You can only accomplish what you believe is possible for
you. And being slim is not impossible!*

Do you use every excuse available to overeat?

Vacation, the wedding, Bar Mitzvah, my birthday, your
birthday, their anniversary. Holidays, picnics, movies,
luncheons, dinners out, dinners in. Nothing in the house to
eat, too much in the house to eat, there's a whole cake and it's
bothering you, it's the last piece of cake and it's bothering

you. You're lonely, you have too much company, you have too much time on your hands and you're bored, you're too busy and have to eat when you can. You're married and he drives you nuts, you're a widow and he was your whole life. Your husband isn't affectionate, he's an animal and paws at you all the time. She doesn't mind you being overweight, she never gets off your back. Readers, please write if you have any additional suggestions for Chapter 2 of the *Encyclopedia*.

Do you lie about what and how much you eat?

It's the old "Don't look at me, *I* didn't eat it!" Now let's be serious for just a minute.

1. It seems to be gone.
2. You are overweight.
3. You've got chocolate icing on your mouth.

Anyone who looks at you can see you ate it—and if it wasn't that particular morsel, it sure was thousands of others. You can have on old underwear and it may not show, or have dirty hair and it might not look too bad, but if you're eating everything that's not nailed down, believe me, *it shows!* And who are you lying to, anyway? Lying is an insult against the intelligence of the person you are lying to, and two terrible things usually come of that. First, they stop believing everything you say. But worse, you start believing it. And when you start lying to yourself, kids, it's all over but the shouting.

Until now, when shedding pounds got hard, did you give up easily?

Whenever one of my Slim-U member says to me "B.Z., I quit!", I know *I* haven't failed—it means quitting is a way of life for them. Sure, sometimes they come back, but that's a learned process as much as quitting is. Giving up is like lying—it's a pretty easy habit to acquire. The difference is that losing weight involves two extremely nasty words—hard work. Hey! Nobody said that holding this book and working your eyeballs over it would cause you to lose weight. It's not easy—just possible. Everyone finds that the things you want take hard work. In fact, even getting fat took hard work. Now if you will only put all that weight behind you and work at getting slim, it will work like a charm.

Do you believe you have the ability to succeed this time?

If you don't, just put down this book and head for the nearest fast food restaurant, because you'll never do it if you don't believe. We've all been taught to accept failure like a true soldier—and we've become real Spartans at it. Now failure's easy, but success—that's a new one. It means responsibility, work and self-esteem—and no one teaches that in college. Just think about being successful in being slim. Of course if you don't *like* being slim, you can always do something about it, right? Over my dead body!

These questions are things I started asking myself as I started getting slim, and with the pounds disappearing, I could be more and more honest. You can do the same. These aren't questions you ask yourself once and then never ponder again. The answers really change as you lose weight. Pick them up once a week and just change the tense of the verb: "Have I been..." Believe me, I still do it. Every day is still a choice for me—whether to stay slim or give in. I haven't completely conquered all twenty yet, either. But little by little, we can all find better consequences in our own truths behind these questions.

8

The Five W's (Who, What, When, Where and Why You're Fat)

First off, let's make certain that we understand each other here. This chapter is *not* a study in Blaming. Blaming is handled in Chapter 10, but there's no use jumping to that section because I don't allow you to blame other people for your being fat in *that* chapter, either. So sit tight and handle one chapter at a time.

In your heart of hearts, you know that as much as you'd like to pass the buck with as much psychological padding as you can, there's absolutely no one who puts food into your mouth forcefully except *you*. The exception to the rule, of course, is feeding cake to your spouse on your wedding day.

Seriously, though, if we better understand the world of our temptations, we'll be better able to fight them off—kind of like taking special care of yourself when the flu is going around. An ounce of prevention is worth about 35 unwanted pounds!

The key to becoming slim is to be aware of the reasons for your overeating.

After reading this chapter, you'll have a much keener sense of how to help yourself. Like guerilla warfare—always be aware of your surroundings.

With Friends Like That...

I swear to you that you will meet someone like the person (or persons) I am about to describe. Once you lose some weight and start feeling pretty good about sashaying down the street (and not causing a traffic jam), you're bound to run into someone like this...

"Oh, B.Z., how *delightful* to see you. Why, I almost didn't recognize you."

(At this point, you begin to beam a good deal.)

"But what kind of diet have you been on? You look *dreadful*. So drawn—it makes your eyes look immense. I guess that's because your face is so gaunt."

(Do not attempt to explain your dieting to her. She doesn't want to know. But here's a lesson in the English language: "drawn" means that your waist is showing—and quite admirably. "Your eyes look immense" —natch! Who ever knew what color they were when they were slits peeking over a couple of fat cheeks.)

"Oh, come on, B.Z. I think it's about time you gave up this dieting nonsense! Here we are in the best ice cream store in town and what do you order—a diet cola! One sundae won't hurt."

(You must remember that from now on, the phrase "this one little bit won't hurt" applies only to tetanus shots and haircuts. This control of yours is clearly killing her. Never have you gotten such sweet revenge from this bitch. You've won!)

"With you on this crazy dieting kick, Bill and Bilinda must be on the verge of starvation. Really, B.Z., the way you feed your family these diet meals, you should be reported to the Society for the Prevention of Cruelty to Children."

(Ha! Cruelty to Children? The way this broad stuffs cheesecake and french fries down her kids' throats, she's lucky they don't roll to school. What will she think forty years from now when the doctor is telling her kids they show signs of heart disease due to poor eating habits? And when her daughter isn't asked to the Senior Prom because no one wants to date a fat girl, will she remember all those cakes and cookies with love? When her fat son is turned down for the job he wants, will Mom's apple pie make up for the pay-check? All that and widowed at 40 because her husband died—at 45 pounds overweight—of cardiac arrest? Now *there's* cruelty for you...)

"Really, B.Z., you look a little peaked and worn down. You should really put a little meat on those bones."

(I've taken so much meat off so many bones over the years that the thought is staggering—all I can see is one of those picked-clean dinosaurs in the museum.)

Anyway, the person described in this hypothetical conversation is *not* a friend. A real friend is someone who wants you to look and feel good, and will help you with your fight with the Battle of the Bulge. The moment you see that dim gleam of green light in their eyes, watch out! There is no underestimating jealousy and envy. Aside from that, your control just goes to show them how much willpower and self-esteem they have themselves. Even if they're slim, your awareness and hold on yourself will hit them like a lead balloon. And lastly, there's always the fear of having someone surpass you. Friends vying for jobs, attention, lovers, *any-thing*, will see you as a threat—and it will be plain to see your feelings about yourself through your demeanor and self-pride. People will see a bigger you than you ever were—but it won't be weight, it will be an aura as big as the room you're in.

So as I say, there's no blaming anyone for being over-weight except yourself, but people in your life like our supposed "friend"—whether they be mother, wife, the Satur-day night pot luck group, your bridge club, *anyone* who tries to force feed you—believe me, they'll make it hard.

Look out for your feelings, not theirs! You'll feel better slim!

I Was Never Tempted by a Turnip

Or a beet, or a few brussel sprouts. But put me in the same room as a plate of brownies—look out! When I ask my Slim-U friends "What kind of food tempts you?" they invariably say "Everything." But when you think about it, it's really not true. But from the look of things, it seems you've put yourself in some rather tempting situations, doesn't it? Let's try to pin down *what* happens each day to cause us to put on the pounds...

As I've said before, no one needs to carry around a little calorie booklet and a calculator to tell them what they can or cannot eat. *Everybody* on the face of the earth *knows* that eating chocolate cake is not quite the same as chomping on a carrot. In fact, don't remind me...anyway chocolate cake or no, it's not so much what you eat as how much. And only you truly know—if you can keep track—how much you're eating.

But how do we zoom in on the whats in our overeating and try to control them? First, put yourself in this situation. You're in a restaurant, and the waiter tells you that the chef has prepared a new, special dish and he'd like everybody to try just a small portion of this food for some feedback. Now, we have here two of the most delightful words in the English language: "free" and "food." Put them both together and you'll have the world at your door. Anyway, absolutely everyone at the table jumps at the chance to try the New Dish—until they hear that it's sweetbreads. Beef Wellington, si; sweetbreads, no! This, indeed, is an easy way to determine what strikes your fancy—clearly, the temptation is not always there.

The best thing to do, then, is make a list. Think of the fattening foods you really crave and write them down. Now, every time you go off to the supermarket, check that list and make sure none of the items is on your shopping list. Buy only what you need and don't start wandering around the aisles of the supermarket. When you start getting in control of yourself, you'll be less apt to trek to a corner store just to pick up that illegal munchie. Step #1 is just to *keep it out of your reach!*

As for preparing food, I've found a way that's good for me, and I think might work for you, too. I cook in quantity. If you're making something you're going to dig into while you're creating it, make it threefold. It probably seems like strange logic—this means there's three times as much to cheat with, right? That may be so, but making it once instead of three times gives you only one chance to cheat instead of three. Freeze what you can and *get out of the kitchen.* When you thaw batch two and three go busy yourself somewhere else instead of hanging around slicing, chopping and nibbling. Believe me, it's a safe bet.

Another "what" question. What *can* I eat when I'm getting rumbly in the stomach and watching the 11 o'clock news? Prepare yourself a legal snack *ahead of time* when you've still got some sense about you and put it aside. Eat it as close to bedtime as possible, therefore avoiding trouble about wanting a second snack. If you find that you're snacking too early in the evening, try to wait an extra fifteen minutes each evening and build up your stamina.

You'll find lots of suggestions about good foods and meal planning in the appendices of this book that my Slim-U people find helpful. It may sound from the way I'm talking here that I'm keeping the secrets of healthy eating to myself, but that's not true at all. A good dieting regimen is essential, but to lead someone through it step by step (now you may eat a piece of toast, have half a hard-boiled egg at 2:46 P.M.) is not letting the dieter control himself. So, turn to the back for suggestions, but turn to the text for encouragement!

The Worst of Times

Before we take a look at situations that often cause us to overeat, let's take a quick look at your eating patterns. Answer yes or no to these questions:

Am I hungry within two hours after a meal?
Do I snack?
Do I eat more than one helping at mealtimes?
Do I eat more than two helpings?
Do I skip meals more than once a week?
Do I need to lose fifteen pounds or more?
Are my meals eaten without regard to balance and nutrition?
If I snack, do I choose high-calorie foods?
Once I start eating—whether at a meal or snacking, is it difficult to stop until I am stuffed?
Is my "sweet tooth" or other particular craving more important to me than my health, fitness and looks?

If you answered "yes" to more than two of these questions, your eating pattern is probably not a good one. As a matter of fact, a yes answer to any question is good reason to look into that particular eating habit—and that goes for overweight *and* slim people.

You may have honest "no" answers to most of these, and can't understand why you're overweight. Surprisingly enough, just one bad habit regarding when and how you eat can make all the difference in whether you've got some extra pounds on you or not. And bad eating habits are the fat person's downfall.

But other than specific times of day, we all know there are times when certain kinds of stress seem to lead us to the refrigerator like a sleepwalker. Face it, fat and thin people alike probably have the same amount of stress. The thing with overweight people is that we'll *create* a nervewracking situation if we have to. Then we find ourselves head-first in the trough, drowning our sorrows. Let's pinpoint some of these situations so we can see them coming next time—some of them aren't so easy to spot.

Remember, being aware of your reasons behind your actions is the key!

Boredom is a tricky one. God invented television so we could watch that when we're bored instead of eat, but the human mind is so clever it figured out how to do both at once. Many people don't understand how terribly stressful it can be to be bored. If you've got a lot of pent-up energy and nothing to do with it, sure as hell you're going to head for the kitchen. It's the same thing that happens when someone stops smoking—almost everyone will tell you they've gained weight. But nine times out of ten they just plug in another mindless thing to do with their hands, and that's certain to translate to a cupcake. Always try to have some little project going—a bit of needlepoint, a fix-it job you've been putting off, a letter you've simply got to write. Away from home, maybe a magic cube. That will certainly keep your mind off food—and everything else.

The self-image problem, as another example of stress, can be a vicious circle and takes a great deal of picking oneself up by the bootstraps. You feel terrible about something within yourself—whether real or imagined—and you start right into some heavy eating. Again, what you feel about yourself that's making you so miserable may be a complete fallacy—*you might invent it in order to eat*. But whether it is a reality or not, it seems real at the time, and there's nothing worse than feeling bad about yourself. We all know that however much our loved ones try to show us our good points and assure us of our worth, nobody can accomplish that long-term except the person in question. Here's the scenario—correct me if I'm wrong, but I'd stake a fortune on this one; it's happened to me a few times too, you know. You feel like maybe you're a tad overweight (or fifty pounds—it really doesn't matter). Who is your only savior? Who can make you feel better, at least for a few moments? Well, at this point, it's not you. But a sundae might do it, or a coffee cake ...So, here we go again, off on a binge, only to realize the minute it's over that you've been your own worst enemy one more time...

I'd like to share one of my most amazing Slim-U experiences with you—a story of a woman who took so much abuse upon herself that she seemed to be spiraling downward so fast that no one could catch up to even try and help her. Not too long ago, Susan was a waddling, huffing, puffing mass of human flesh who weighed 406 pounds. Her life seemed over and she was frantically digging a grave with her fork. As is often the case, Susan's problems were not just physical, but psychological as well. She had no self-esteem and no dignity, and she had been trying to fight the battle of the bulge and was losing ground rapidly.

Susan had gotten herself into a horrendous marriage, but she stayed with it eating her way through the days. She had no job, four children and an enormous body. Sue began to believe she deserved the misery she was experiencing.

The first time Susan walked up to the scales at Slim-U, she locked her eyes with mine and with desperation and determination whispered, "Please help me, I can't take this fat any longer. My doctor told me to go home and kiss my children goodbye because at the rate I was going I wouldn't live to raise them." Then she began to cry. Well, we both knew it would be all-out war to change a lifetime of hiding food, lying about what you've eaten and all the while wanting to be slim more than anything else in the world. When she didn't show up at a meeting, I'd call her and she'd start to explain why she was absent and I told her outright that she was speaking to the world's biggest liar on the subject of weight and it was foolish to try to outfox a fox. There were a lot of angry words between Susan and me, but one thing never changed—we had a mutual love for each other and a mighty enemy to slay. I'm happy and proud to announce to the world that Susan, at this writing, has lost over 260 pounds, and before you read this book, she will be *slim*. But hear it from Susan herself—this is an excerpt of a letter she wrote to me:

Dear B.Z.,

Today I am reborn; no more bad marriage, my children are growing and happier than they have ever been. You and I and Slim-U have come a long way together. What all of us have shared at Slim-U is the joy of a special love for each other and ourselves, transcended only by the ultimate joy of losing weight and being in control of our lives. Barbara, you move mountains (I know, I was one of them) by helping others to rebuild attitudes about themselves.

As I progress in the joy of my accomplishments, they are topped only by the look in my mirror or in the eyes of my children and friends. I am becoming the type of woman that once I only dared to dream of. My life is filled with more excitement now than even a box of cookies, and that says it all.

Love you, B.Z.
Susan

Well, I'm afraid for all of you who might have come this far looking for miracles, Susan has said it all—no miracle, *just control of yourself.* I think most of us will agree—Susan's problems make ours look like a word we've always treasured—miniscule.

But there are other problems we can blame weight gain on, if we try hard enough. How about the worries of a new career, problems in love, moving our home, sickness—our own or someone else's—kids leaving the nest, financial woes, divorce, menopause (male or female!)—and a score of other things. Do you truly think you're the only one who has these problems? There aren't any 90 pound weaklings with creditors knocking at their doors? C'mon! Lift yourself out of your self-pity for a moment and maybe you'll get the same sort of overview Susan did. When she saw that her life looked like Hiroshima, she took the only step she could—she started picking up the pieces. She sure made my problems seem a lot smaller. Don't you think so, too?

Danger Zones

Ah, a lesson in geography. We will start with *kitchen*, from the old Greek word meaning "Fatso." It is so often said that fat women are great cooks, but the truth is, fat women are great eaters. They may be great cooks, too, but the percentages there are pretty damn good considering how much time they spend in the kitchen. In the kitchen not cooking, that is. Look, there are scores of cookbooks that tell you how to cook great recipes in under an hour. Make it now, bake it later doesn't mean stuff everything in sight down your throat in between, it means do something *constructive* in between. Keep busy! The only reason we spend so much time in the sacred kitchen is because we've made it our lifeline—and the kitchen is a terrible lifeline. It can't possibly help us at all. They make our lives hell, and we treat them, well, like the Garden of Eatin'.

Not to despair. Of course there's a solution—should you choose to accept it.

Stay out of the kitchen as much as possible!

Really try to eat only at mealtimes. That's not quite as hard as you think if you help yourself out. Use phone extensions *outside* the kitchen. Set your stove timer indicating when you absolutely must enter the kitchen to prepare for the next meal—and don't jump the gun. Eat only when you're seated—with placemat, utensils and napkin. (No, I'm not trying to make you into a society matron, just trying to unmake the savage!) No eating while standing, leaning over the sink or with the head conveniently tucked into the fridge. Beginning now, try to excel in another room. I suggest the bedroom—unless you find that less interesting than the TV room...

Eating alone is also a real danger zone. When I was a kid, my mother used to say "Never do anything you'd be ashamed to do in front of a crowd." I wish she had said "Don't eat anything you wouldn't eat in front of a crowd." Not that I can blame her, folks, but at least I can pass that advice along to you today. As most of you do, I did my most destructive eating while by my lonesome. Again, no matter how many times we might say we weren't aware of it, deep down we know how we wait for our cohabitants to go to bed, run an errand, answer the phone, *anything*. Lots of times we'll have food hidden everywhere for every occasion. And rid the house of cute little candy dishes filled with the goodies of the particular season, etc. Your guests and family never really see much of them anyway, do they? Wonder how I know all these tricks? Well where the hell do you think I've been all these years?!

I asked a friend of mine recently who had gotten control of herself and lost a good deal of weight how she passed up ice cream for sale on the streets when the vendors were practically begging you to try it (I was having a hard time myself). "Well," she said, "I try to stand half way between the ice cream wagon and the fruit stand. Then, for five or ten minutes, I watch the people who go to the ice cream man and the ones who go to the fruit stand. After observing the clientele at both, I haven't made a wrong decision yet." Comprende?

When you go to a party, just remember, it's not your last party *or* your last plate of ice cream, but when put in a situation like this which you know is going to drive you crazy, just make sure you eat beforehand. If you don't trust yourself at the party, bring something legal of your own along. The last thing to worry about is that the other guests will catch on that you're dieting. Believe me, they've already caught on that you're fat, they'll do nothing but applaud you when they see you're trying to beat it. And you should feel proud that you're manifesting your self-worth to them by showing them up front that you know you're worth *more* than your weight in gold.

Vacations, you'll say next. How do I overcome getting fat on a vacation? First of all, answer this question honestly. Is your first reaction to a vacation "Ah, I've waited all year for this. I'm going to eat whatever I want!" You haven't been eating what you want all year? I couldn't have told by looking at you. How many years more will you run out and buy a few overblousy things at the last minute. And years when you couldn't find a bathing suit to fit you? Years when you wouldn't ski because you couldn't see your feet? Like to do that again? Vacations should be—and can be—one of the easiest times to diet, *if you let it*. That means not taking along a supply of quarters for vending machines, and ordering sensibly (fruit for dessert, please) in restaurants (remember, people are watching you!). Take this book along so you can refer to the Slim-U program when in doubt. Take your fattest picture of yourself and leave it on top of the clothes in your suitcase—every time you open it you'll be reminded. With a little luck and some stamina, you'll be able to fit a hell of a lot more clothes in that suitcase next vacation!

I hate to sound like a bore, but again, the trick is to be *aware*. Just as we know what foods are highly fattening, we sure as hell know which times we are most susceptible to overeating. And if you really want to lose weight, you've got to prepare in advance for each battle—no surprise attacks—and then charge!

Why Me?

In Chapter 10 we deal with this question in depth, but in short, let me answer it here with great philosophical flourish: *because you overate.* Shocked? Offended? Too bad, toots, that's the whole truth and nothing but the truth. But still, you say that it must be someone or something that made me unhappy enough to overeat. Well, you're right on that point. I truly believe this:

Obesity is the outward sign of an inward illness.

Let me quickly add, a *curable* illness—but an illness nonetheless. But as with any illness, we should concentrate not just on curing it, but on what caused it; then we can dwell on the cause of our illness and make sure it doesn't recur. Overeating is habit-forming, so even if we were to pinpoint our problem right off, we still have to recondition ourselves to eat normally. Like I've said, no miracles. And now that we've uncovered a bit of enemy camouflage in our War with Food, let's slaughter those dragons and move into the positive—how to avoid those tempting times.

9

How to Avoid Overeating

In the previous chapter, we spent some time exploring the various difficulties of being fat and the numerous temptations that befall us at what seems like every turn. As we've discussed, being fat is a choice and ridding yourself of unwanted pounds is a matter of control. Many times, though, it's a hell of a lot easier on us if we have some concrete things or tasks to turn to when that ol' banana split comes a-knockin' at our door. This chapter is one to pick up anytime you feel threatened and need a little strength. It's full of tips on how to otherwise spend your time outside the world of food.

Keeping Busy

The number-one food culprit for so many people is boredom. If you don't work, or are home alone, or if you work on a conveyor belt producing marshmallow eggs, you are bound to be bored. Overeating is a normal hobby to pick up. It's easy, no bother cleaning up after yourself, and you can do it alone. The only drawback is that it makes you fat. Oh, you'd noticed that? Well then, perhaps the idea is to keep yourself busy with other things every time your fingers start getting itchy. Try some of these—you don't have to be training for the Olympics for these activities, and even the tiniest bit of self-improvement (remember the one pushup?) always, *without fail*, makes you feel better.

Walking.

It is still possible to do it even in this age of technology, and get this, *you can do it without the aid of holding a shopping cart!* I know it sounds wild, but it's not so bad. Think of all the times each day you jump into your car to go a block or two—just to mail a letter or get to the corner store. There's no reason for it and chances are the few extra minutes you take to walk instead of drive will have a surprisingly calming effect on you.

Simple exercises.

No need to overdo. If you can't touch your toes yet, don't worry, you will. For now, do a couple of sit-ups, securing your feet under something if you have to. Or stretch your arms out at your sides and twist your torso as far each way as you can—it's good for the tummy. Everyone knows some simple exercises; just do a few every time your mind turns to eating. You'll be helping yourself doubly.

Bike riding.

With the new ten-speeds, it's a cinch. You haven't forgotten how, I promise you. Borrow your kid's bike and zip around the block a few times. Don't attempt the hilly sections of town first. Remember, for you lazy fatties, you're sitting down while you're bike riding.

Gardening.

This is not overtaxing—it's relaxing, you can taste the fruits of your efforts (don't plant any pecan pie seeds) and it's cost-efficient. And again, you're getting outdoors, which is about as far away from the refrigerator as you can get.

There are other things you can do, too, which don't involve simple exercises as the activities I just mentioned all do. The ideas I just mentioned are helpful because they can all be enjoyed in the amount of time you want to allot to them—a few minutes or a couple of hours. But you may find that you have an inordinate amount of time on your hands, and this makes you feel like there's nothing else to do but dig in. You may need more involving projects.

Do-it-yourself.

Why not? You've got the time, teach yourself a few new tricks. Get one of those all encompassing how-to manuals and get to work fixing all the things that are too miniscule to call in a repairman for, but have been driving you crazy. If you find you're not the Have-Wrench-Will-Travel type, what about needlework, sketching, calligraphy? There are so many interesting things we've promised ourselves we'd learn, and now's the time!

Writing letters.

Here's another lost art like walking. People love a telephone call but *adore* getting a letter. Besides, you don't have to write a letter in the kitchen, and I'll bet that's where you make your phone calls. And for an all-out terrific time on a day when you feel particularly susceptible to binging, pay the bills! There's no greater feeling. Well, hardly...

Volunteer work.

I know it sounds old-fashioned, but giving up a few hours a week isn't going to kill you, and what can be better than making someone else feel good at the same time you're making yourself feel good?

Self-improvement.

Now that you're going to be beautiful and svelte, you're going to want to be gorgeous all over, right? And the beauty of working on improvements on other parts of your body is that it doesn't take time like losing weight does. Get a new haircut, a manicure, a pair of new shoes. Just because you can't be thin tomorrow is no reason not to start preparing for the day you are!

There's lots more you can do—you don't need me to think things up for you. Just make sure you do something positive to reinforce the fact that you're changing your life for the better. And while you're at it, give yourself a pat on the back for staying away from food!

Treating Yourself

No, not with a reward of a cupcake! We've been so used to rewarding ourselves with food when we think we've done something to deserve a treat that cupcakes, french fries and another slice of pumpkin bread are the first things we think of. After all, they rarely give medals to civilians, right? So what else is there?

Well, the first thing to change is your attitude about rewards. From here on in, we do not wait until we've done something we feel Dan Rather needs to know about before we get to treat ourselves. From this moment forward, we will treat ourselves when we feel like it. Aha! I can see the guilt creeping into your eyes. Treating myself when I've done nothing special? Heresy! Well, tell me why the hell not. Isn't each day tough enough that you deserve for someone to come along and say "Hey, B.Z., you're doing one swell job at living." And who does? No one! So do it yourself. If you're truly not cheating on your diet, you should be saving a couple of bucks a day. Don't spend it on someone else—you were never that selfless before. Buy something for yourself that you've been wanting for a long time. This is the time to try the fancy new hairdresser in town or buy the new bestseller *before* it comes out in paperback. Live it up! No one else can pay better attention to you than you can.

Avoiding Guilt and Frustration

A lot of us have been brought up by parents who use guilt as a weapon in childraising. And boy, does it work! In fact, it works so well that by the time we're at the age of reason we can feel guilty all by ourselves with only the teeniest bit of provocation.

There is absolutely no value in guilt. Guilt isn't like a hot stove—you'll keep doing it over and over again no matter how much it hurts if it's worth it to you. Guilt induces guilt, so if you cheat on your diet and manage to convince yourself that you've blown the whole diet forever, you'll run to the refrigerator to drown yourself in your guilt. Real guilt comes when you know you have a legitimate reason for feeling guilty: you constantly overeat and lie about it, you're an alcoholic or a kleptomaniac. You feel guilt then because you know you're doing something wrong. The solution is obvious, though not necessarily simple. Stop. You'll never stop feeling guilty until you stop doing whatever it is that isn't right for you.

Now cheating on a diet should not be a guilt-inducing trip. At the point where you snitch a little food and go into a fit of depression over it, you have lost control of yourself. Not because you cheated, but because at this point you are saying "Look, I've failed again. I just can't do it alone. Someone has to help me." Well who the hell else is going to do it for you short of straightjacketing you? If you feel guilty about something you've done, chalk it up to experience and try to avoid doing it again. There's nothing you can do after a fall but pick yourself up.

There will surely be times on your diet when you are frustrated. Either you expected to lose more than you did this week or you've done terrificly and no one noticed—something's bound to come up. And not everyone, especially if they're uncomfortably overweight, can take out their frustrations by playing a few sets of tennis. But frustration, if you let it, will immobilize you. You must face it at once and do something to get it out of your system and lessen its importance.

Now there's no one who agrees with you more on what it is that has frustrated you and how unfair the whole situation is. Naturally, that person is you. I find that the best way to handle this is to sit right down and write myself a letter, as the song goes. Be careful not to degrade yourself—you don't need that, but be firm and honest. Talk about *why* you're frustrated, how real the situation is. If you've blown it out of proportion, admit it: no one else is reading the letter. Talk about how you're going to change your plan of attack, remind yourself how much this diet means to you. Let it all out—say how tough it is, how much it hurts, but *always* wind up (even if it takes a ream of paper!) saying that you know you can beat it!

Talk to your friends. You don't have to tell them why you're down in the dumps, and they're not interested in hearing your "No one loves me" spiel. But if you talk with someone who really cares about you, they will inevitably end up reminding you how terrific you are. Friends aren't around to say "Don't eat that" but to let you know that "You deserve it and you owe it to yourself."

Again, when you're frustrated is one of the best times to do something for yourself. It makes you feel absolutely wicked for some reason, and that feels great. Write up a new resume, sew a dress a size too small, call a person or prospective client you've been wanting to meet. Prove to yourself that you really are on top and can do something you've been avoiding. It will enhance your belief that you can do anything, including being thin!

When you feel frustrated, remember these three things:

> frustration is a time-waster;
> frustration is a guilt-inducing emotion;
> frustration is a self-pitying technique.

Bowing to frustration is just another way of saying that you're not giving yourself the chance you deserve. You're punishing yourself and asking for someone else to take control. You're asking for someone to force-feed your diet—and your life.

Overcoming Your Plateaus

The dreaded dieting plateau. What could be worse! All week long my Slim-U members (well, some of them) diet like crazy, never cheat and count the minutes until our next meeting, absolutely sure that they've lost at least three pounds due to their arduous care. Then they get on the scales. No change. Exactly, to the ounce, the same weight they were the week before. Are they outraged? You might say that. All the weeks that they've cheated a little here and there and still lost a pound or two come flooding back to them—not that they can cite these for fear of giving away their indiscretions, but wow, are they ticked off. And who can blame them? You've been honest and God has cheated you out of *at least* two pounds.

I'm making light of it, but that plateau is a drag, because you really don't deserve it. For some reason, the body does catch up with itself and realigns forces before it goes on. Remember, you're fighting your body and it's going to react like anybody else who's threatened—protective. But a plateau never lasts more than about ten days. That's one reason that we encourage weighing-in only once a week at Slim-U. It's plain discouraging to weigh yourself every day. This losing of weight is no miracle, and you can't expect drastic changes every day.

During the time you are at a plateau on your diet— which may occur more than once—is the best time to be rewarding yourself. *You* know you haven't done anything wrong and *I* know you haven't done anything wrong, but someone didn't tell your fat behind. Treat yourself extra special now.

Frustration is also its own plateau. When you get frustrated you come to a dead stop, just as your body does. You've got to make sure that you keep yourself moving in a forward direction. It may be at a snail's pace, but at least you've got the stamina to move on. Always keep your goals reasonable. If you want to lose 50 pounds, and you really believe you will, more power to you. But don't promise yourself that you're going to do it in two months—and try not to think of it as a life-long process either. Be realistic with your goals and you'll not only be pleasantly surprised, you'll be keeping your frustration level down, too.

Let me say one more thing about plateaus. In the real sense of the word, plateau is the goal, a leveling off. Think of it as a point you have finally reached. You can rest there and move on when you're ready. Be thankful that you got there in the first place and remember that it wasn't so long ago that you were way down below that plateau looking up at it with binoculars. Didn't ever think you'd get this far, did you?

Be Your Own Best Friend

Are you sick of hearing this? Are you just about going to throw it up if I say it again? *You are your own best friend.* You're pretty hot. No one else is going to treat you as well as you can treat yourself. In the long run, no one cares about you as much as you do—the applause does stop, even for

Katharine Hepburn. Or maybe I should really be saying that you *can* be your own best friend. From the looks of things now, you've done a hell of a job at being your own worst enemy. Think of the person you like least on this earth. Now if they had a chance to get back at you, what do you think they'd do. First, they add about 73 pounds to your gorgeous body. Then, they'd make you feel awful every day by making you uncomfortable, embarrassed, short of breath and generally unattractive. Then they'd find someone to steal your husband away and cause you to lose your job because it's too expensive to keep you at two desks. And then the children! They'll take the children because of the terrible eating habits you've taught them. One day, you'll wait for them to come home from school to their cupcakes and chocolate milk, and they will never return...

Alright, maybe I got a little carried away, but some of those things are true, aren't they? The part about the 73 pounds and the feeling uncomfortable and unattractive? Just let me ask this one question of you if you don't intend to lose that weight:

Can it get better?

10

Who Made Me Fat? The Real You

So you've noticed you're putting on a few pounds. You just can't understand how it happened, but there it is, the mirror proves it. Obviously *you* didn't have anything to do with it, but some funny telltale signs have become apparent. Check each of these statements that's true for you. Then, tally your score and see if you should be on Fat Albert.

You Know You're Getting Fat When...

You've left your doctor's office in tears more than once during the past six months.

The boy who delivers the groceries has a hernia.

Last time you had a flat tire, a handsome stranger gave you directions to the nearest pay phone.

Your spouse/lover doesn't know your dress size.

Your best friend doesn't know your dress size.

During lovemaking, you find yourself sucking in your tummy.

You have, on occasion, eaten a bowl of ice cream in a closet.

You shower by candlelight—alone.

Your neighbors wait on the landing until you climb the stairs.

You can recite the TV lineup for Saturday night.

Someone gave you a flannel nightgown for Christmas. You've worn it.

Your mother no longer encourages you to clean your plate.

You know how to spell and define "panacea" without the aid of a dictionary.

Suddenly, you despise the salesperson in the sportswear section of your favorite department store.

The chic little French boutique around the corner from your office hasn't had anything that fit you in two years.

You perspire getting dressed.

You like to wear black, navy blue and brown.

Your legs are considerably shorter than they used to be.

Construction workers giggle as you pass.

Now give yourself three points for each true statement:

0–9   You're a skinny person who read this for laughs.
12–24 Have a salad for lunch tomorrow. It's still not too late.
27–36 Jog, don't walk, to the nearest gym.
39–51 Have you ever considered going on a three-week fast?
54–60 Congratulations—you really are an Earth Mother!

Passing the Buck

So you didn't pass the test with flying colors, eh? You're overweight and you can't understand what on earth happened. You've been eating like you always have, maybe a few more snacks to tide you over, but what could it be? Let me dispel some of the usual excuses people use for their obesity.

It's inherited.

That may well be. If your mother was fat and fed you all the same junk she was feeding herself, probably you're from a whole family of blimps. Fat families just come from a long line of poor eating habits. And if your mother was overweight when you were born, you may have had more fat cells in you at birth than some babies. The trick is to keep the fat cells empty.

I have a thyroid problem.

Boy, is that ever a favorite. Most people don't even *know* what a thyroid problem is, but they'll assume that it's their problem if they're overweight. Ask any doctor—one has nothing to do with the other.

I have big bones.

So does Margaux Hemingway. So does Candy Bergen. What they don't have is big fat on those big bones. They seem to manage quite well, those big girls.

I've just been through a divorce.

If people got fat because they've been through a divorce, there would be no Hollywood. Who'd want to look at a whole slew of movies with fat people in them? Divorce is a stressful situation, certainly, but one which we will use as an excuse for our overeating. In a low self-esteem situation that is common in post-divorce months, to nosedive into depression and eating too much is common. Notice I say common—people pick themselves up by their bootstraps every day after a divorce; but they don't all get fat in the meantime. It's just one way of punishing ourselves further for what we see as a failure on our part. Try to think about now, not the past.

I just had a baby.

So did Charo. Apparently, though, the doctors didn't keep the secrets of exercising from her like they have from you.

I had a hysterectomy.

This is my all-time favorite, and you wouldn't believe how many women tell this one with a straight face. Just tell me how it is that someone has parts taken *out* of them and that makes them fatter.

There are countless more excuses, of course, but they only get more ridiculous as we go on. All I'm trying to say is that you can pass the buck as much as you want, but you might as well post a sign on you that says, "The Fat Stops Here." Because that's the truth, isn't it? I think it says something that no matter who or how you place the blame, the results always show up on you. I'm afraid, dear hearts, that we've got nobody to blame but ourselves.

"Ask Anybody—I Never Cheat!"

If you tell me right now that you've never said this before, I am going to call you one hell of a liar. Luckily, I can't see your face, so you don't have to look an old pro like me in the eye. No one ever cheats. That's how we all got so fat—by not cheating. Or people tell themselves that the way they're feeding themselves is sensible for their particular predicament. Someone's bound to tell you as you catch them with a pb & j sandwich in their mitt at 9:30 A.M. that they saw a friend in the hospital last night who got sick, poor thing, and had no extra weight to fall back on. Most chubbies I've seen had better be cautious. If they ever get sick and fall back on those fat asses it will take them a week to stop bouncing.

Oh, and most heavy people, don't you know, could easily qualify for a medical degree. Without any test or determination by a doctor, they know that they've got hypoglycemia (low blood sugar). Of course this sounds good because these experts think the only way to counteract this serious medical problem is to eat lots of sweets and bring their blood sugar back to normal. "I felt my blood sugar go way down Thursday, so I had two chocolate bars, a piece of coffee cake and a glazed donut and, thank God, I started to feel better immediately." Funny that these geniuses have never heard of *hyper*-glycemia.

Or how about the fat lady who says "You've no idea how I hate being fat, and I'd really like to lose weight, but my husband gets really mad when I start losing—he likes me this way." Now, there's not a weight group director in the world who can tackle that one without coming out the loser. We know what she says is true because who does her husband look at on the beach? That's right, his eyes wander over every fat woman in a bikini, and that's why *Playboy* uses all fat girls for their centerfold. A big, nude female with rolls of fat really turns guys on and sells lots of magazines.

Hey, how about "I'm a slow loser." (The way you eat, it's no wonder!) "Of course, you've no way of knowing this, but I've been on every diet known to man, and it's next to impossible for me to lose. Let me give you an example—once I went on a skim milk and banana diet. Do you know how I suffered? Six bananas a day was all the solid food I ate. I'm probably the only human being alive that can peel a banana with one hand. And after three weeks of this monkeying around (ugh!), I only lost one pound! Then I tried a water diet. That was agony. I couldn't leave the house without knowing a bathroom was nearby. After a month, I lost two pounds! Next I tried my own idea—eat less and sleep more. I started staying in bed later in the morning and by so doing, I delayed breakfast until 10 A.M. By then I was weak from hunger, so I had a very large breakfast. By the time I finished and cleaned up, it was lunchtime. Having completed that task, I figured it was time to have a snack, take a sleeping pill, and call it a day. I gained three pounds! So you can see, it's clearly impossible for me to lose weight."

Here's one that really blows our cover. "I really eat very little—if you don't believe me, ask my husband." You've got to admit, that's a brave statement. After all, your husband would certainly know if you were going around eating fattening things. Ah, friends, we are so crafty and quick that even God isn't sure! Do you think my husband knew that every night when I took off my bra it was full of cookie crumbs? Are you kidding? Who but a fat lady—a fat lady who cheats, that is—would even think of hiding cookies in her bra and eating them as she walks around the house?

Say, aren't those drive-in windows at the fast food places great for not cheating? Just sit in the parking lot some day and see your friends drive through. A short stop at the window, and then around the building. Park way in the back. Why? Well, you've heard of a quickie, haven't you? Well, to a fat lady, this is a quickie. A little something to hold her over till she gets to the supermarket.

Fat people eat in the strangest places. Locked bathrooms, back seats of cars, closets, laundry rooms, parking lots, under a towel at the beach, in a pitch black room—almost anyplace except at a table, in front of people. And these are only my own secret cheating places—I'll bet you've got a few you're keeping to yourself.

Have you ever met a friend in a coffee shop at two o'clock in the afternoon? Doesn't she always tell you that she was so busy shopping that she forgot all about lunch, and has just realized that she hasn't eaten? That will be the day. You and I know that she ate lunch at eleven o'clock—of course, that was only to beat the rush. Funny, thin people never make excuses for eating, and fat people never stop.

How about all the cute little cakes and stuff that we buy for the kids lunches and then eat ourselves? No one would ever think you were buying goony-looking things like that for anyone over the age of twelve. Oh, how many times have you wanted to die when one of your big-mouthed kids shouted, "Hey, someone stole my Mounds bar!" There you stand in utter helplessness, knowing full well that you are the somebody being referred to, and praying that no one will guess. Even when the fight begins, and you are an accomplice to your kids' sibling rivalry, you sit rooted to your chair, not daring to admit that the Phantom has struck again.

For five blissful years I had two marvelous Phantoms in my life—the famous Dillon kids from next door. Whenever anything was eaten and I was questioned, I simply said that Mike and Denise had been playing at our house and must have eaten it themselves. If those kids had really eaten all the junk I blamed on them, they would have been ear-to-ear pimple—instead of me being wall-to-wall fat!

There's another handy routine we have that is really quite sensible. It's called getting it out of the house. It's a well-known fact that when you have a lot of fattening food in the house, the temptation to eat it is sometimes too great. So the best thing to do is get it out of the house. But how? We could put it down the garbage disposal, but that's a terrible waste, and with all the hungry people in the world, it would be a sin. Now if there's one thing we fatties don't want to be held accountable for, it's a food sin. We could give it to someone thin and let them finish it for us, but no, those damn thin people always say "Oh, no, not for me, thanks, I'm trying to lose weight," or "Oh, I couldn't, I just finished dinner about two hours ago and I'm so full I can hardly move." Or the most maddening answer of all, which brings out a genuine killer instinct in fat people—"I'm not hungry." What the hell does that mean? I didn't ask you if you were hungry, I asked you if you wanted a piece of cake. They should know that that has nothing to do with hunger.

Hey, how about giving it to the kids? Couldn't you just go for their throats when they screw up their cute little faces and say, "Yecch, it's too sweet and gooey for me." Why not try a small piece on the dog, and if he eats it, you can feed him the rest. Humph, who expected that old fleabag to sniff, turn up his nose and walk away? Oh well, that just leaves you. God knows you tried, but now there's only one solution—you'll have to eat it yourself. Now don't jump to conclusions. I know what you're thinking—"Here she goes again." Not true. I'm only getting it out of the house so tomorrow I can start on my diet. It's not cheating. No, sir. In fact, I never cheat, you can ask anybody. Well, that is, almost anybody.

Defining Your Fat Type

Now that we know you are indeed the culprit and cause of your obesity, you should be aware of your fat type. Don't tell me you don't know what that is! It's kind of like a blood type—everybody has one. Pointing the finger at your weakness isn't very pleasant, I know, but being aware of your actions is crucial to solving your eating problems. Let's explore some of the fat types.

I belong to the first group—*Closet Eaters*. We never eat much in front of people in a restaurant, so it goes something like this. "Waitress, I'd like my fish broiled without butter, please substitute the string beans for the french fries, and will you tell the kitchen to please hold the dressing? I have my own. Oh, and do you have any diet soda?" Now everyone at the table is highly impressed with our determination to stick to our diet when faced with such unbelievable temptation. Of course, they don't know that since lunch we've eaten two bologna sandwiches, two handfuls of potato chips, a leftover cupcake from our kid's lunchbox, a small piece of coffee cake, a piece of toast with butter and jelly and half a candy bar which had been almost forgotten at the bottom of our pocketbook. We closet eaters are a mystery to our friends. They can't figure out how we got so fat. They'll swear they've never seen us eat a fattening thing—and heaven knows they never have!

Closet eaters always need someone to back them up, so they're constantly saying "I'm a very small eater, right dear?" Naturally, he thinks you are, and swears to God you hardly eat at all. In all the years we've been married my husband has only ever seen me eat three carrots, two apples and a handful of lettuce. Bet he wonders where $90 worth of groceries go every week, though. Closet eaters also pray a lot. We keep praying that our mates and family will have to go someplace so we can get at the food. From the time Bill leaves to get the newspaper and returns, I can eat out two closets and a large refrigerator and stand there like an angel upon his return. Yes, sir, if you don't believe me, ask my husband.

Group Two is the *Talk Me Into It* Group. Picture this. Thin person: "Oh, look, they have strawberry shortcake, let's have some." Fat lady: "Oh, I really shouldn't, I'm trying to stay on a diet." Hear the word no anywhere? We'll say "I shouldn't" and "I'm trying," but you'll notice the absence of words like "No thank you, I don't care for any." As soon as we announce that we're on a diet, this invites all our friends to feel sorry for us, and we know it. That's why we tell everybody right away— so we can have some help jumping on and off the fatwagon, preventing us from staying straight. The Talk Me into Its are believers of the moment. Whatever they want to hear from a friend, they'll hear—especially if it's "Oh, please join me in a plate of spaghetti. You can start your diet tomorrow."

Group three—*The Calorie Counters*. This type wouldn't dream of leaving the house without her handy little calorie counting book that she picked up at the checkout counter. First, she'll grab the menu in one hand, Diet Bible in the other. Let's see—a chicken breast is 155 calories. That's good. A serving of string beans, uh huh, a glass of tomato juice for an appetizer. Gee, that's great so far, the whole meal only comes to "x" calories. Hey, what's this? Spaghetti and meat balls is only 356. Two slices of Italian bread, add butter, two glasses of wine and cream of celery soup as a starter. Wow, I can afford to eat this if I just don't eat anything else all day. Ha! Are you acquainted with fat chance?

Are you part of the *Dessert Group?* You always order fish because it's not fattening—lobster with drawn butter or something breaded and deep-fried is okay. No potatoes, drinks or bread, though. But what no one at the table knows is that you've already memorized the dessert list. You've spent the whole meal changing your mind three times about what to order, and now, the chocolate cake has won out. And everyone at the table agrees that you're entitled to some enjoyment after all you've passed up.

Perhaps you're part of the *You Deserve a Break Today Group.* This generous soul will take all her children and anyone else's to the fast food joint of their choice. She lets the kids order super-deluxe burgers, milkshakes, fries and fruit pies. Now, she selects a table all the way in the back to be less conspicuous. On the way to the table she manages a few fries from each bag and several huge swigs of milkshake to wash them down. She finishes her own food almost as soon as she is seated. She knows that she who hesitates is lost.

Watch those kids closely, now, because there's always some wise guy who tries to finish his entire burger. You've got to keep hurrying the kids along because they can't eat fast and tend to lose interest in food when they're rushed. Sooner or later (usually fairly soon), she'll eat all the remains of the burgers and fries that the nasty kids have left when we all know children in India are starving. A really altruistic woman.

Last but not least is the most interesting group of all, the *It's Always Something Group.* They never use the same excuse twice, yet they always seem to get away with it. If it goes with the meal and I'm paying for it, you bet I'm going to eat it. Oh, I wish we hadn't come here—they specialize in chocolate mousse and you know I can't resist that. Did you know today is my anniversary, birthday, the first time I've seen my sister in two years, the first day of spring, my last day to bowl, my grandniece's graduation, my grandson's first day at school, the 20th anniversary of D-Day, the last time I'll see my sister for two years, the last day of summer, Alexander Graham Bell's birthday, and I don't give a good gaddamn, *I'm eating it!*

Exploring Your Past Mistakes

See yourself in any of those people? I sure do. I've used all those excuses more than once, believe me. But you can change. Be aware of your past mistakes and try to turn yourself around, slowly but surely. Rome wasn't built in a day, and just because you look like the Coliseum right now doesn't mean you can't look like Sophia Loren in the near future.

I think by now you know that I'm a great believer in lists. And I think that the greatest way to be aware of your past mistakes is to stare them in the face. Since you can't carry this book around everywhere you go, it's good to make your own private lists of your particular trouble spots. For example, make a list of five places you should stay away from—the five that most give you a temptation fit. They might be the ice cream section of the supermarket, Louie's Pasta Parlor, the corner bakery, vending machines, etc. As you get better at conquering these, add more, a few at a time.

As we've said, sometimes your friends are not the best people to trust with your diet. If you find that some of your friends are really troublemakers for your diet, avoid meeting them for lunch or other places where food's the object of the visit. Talk to them on the phone, if you must, until you've got enough stamina to see them in a more tempting situation. Don't hurt their feelings by telling them why you're avoiding them—believe me, they won't understand. Just make yourself scarce for awhile.

Here's the tough one. Make a list of the ten things you commonly eat that you shouldn't. They are now off your Things I'm Allowed to Eat List. However, jot down on the back of the no-no list some tasty things that are legal. Turn to that when you're tempted. I know all these lists make us sound like morons, but they really work. We need blinders on sometimes to keep us aware of our goals. We'll get by with a little help from ourselves, to change the song a bit.

Believe me, folks, there will come a day when some truly amazing occurrences will happen, ones that are exactly the opposite of the situations we mentioned at the beginning of this chapter—and they bring a directly opposing emotion— sheer joy.

You Can Tell You're Getting Slim When...

You stuff your bra to fill the cups.
You don't have to lie down to zip your slacks.
The postman hand-delivers your mail.
Your hip bones stick out past your stomach.
Your purple stretch marks turn pink.
Your husband fires his young secretary.
Your kids put their arms around you...*all* the way around you.
You wear a bathing suit in the light of day.
You weigh yourself in public.
The smell of peanut butter makes you sick.
You say "I don't want any cake"—and mean it.
Your husband buys you a see-through nightie—and you parade around in it.
A friend's husband blows in your ear—and you don't blow back.
You buy a new dress with the leftover grocery money.
You give your old clothes to a fat friend.
You stand in front of a mirror in the nude and you don't turn away.
You read *I Left My Fat Behind* for the fun of it.

It's no dream. Your day will come with a little stamina and a lot of love for the most important person in your life— *you!*

11

B.Z.'s Slim-Down

I almost wanted to start this chapter by calling it a round-up of all the things we've discussed and learned from the pages of this book plus our own experiences. It then occurred to me that this was perhaps a highly negative word for a bunch of fatties whose goal it is to lose weight and really leave their fat behind. So what's the opposite of a round-up? What else! A slim-down! Remember the Friday afternoon round-ups on *The Mickey Mouse Show* when all the little Mouseketeers would put on their cowboy outfits? Well, let's lay aside them weapons of eclairs and gumdrops and gather 'round for a Slim-Down of what you, me and some of my Slim-U members have learned about our shoot-out with fat.

Unless you're an inveterate mystery reader, you've probably read the rest of this book and haven't snuck a look to the final chapter (as if skipping all the previous ones would make you automatically thin if you just read the final chapter). Well, whether you've been fighting fat for a while and used this book as a guideline, or whether you've read this straight through for help and confidence, you're most likely still fighting fat. Reading *I Left My Fat Behind* shouldn't be a one time thing—keep it available to remind yourself that you'd better stay on the straight and narrow if you want to stay slim. We all know that it's really hell to be fat. And the fatter we are, the heller it gets.

If you've been waiting to find out what it's like to be *fit* instead of *fat*, the answer is to combine the pages of this book with a closed mouth and an open mind—an infallible recipe. You'll feel better all the way around—what there *is* to get around. I *guarantee* you that you will feel better about yourself mentally, because you'll know you're in control. People will treat you differently, too, for the same reason. They will realize that you care about yourself and your self-image. You're going to look like a likeable person to like!

Physically, of course, taking your excess weight off will make a world of difference in your life. For those of us who have longed to get on the tennis court, swim a few laps or jog in the crisp early morning, being slim can make our lives totally different and much more enjoyable than they have been in a long time. And for those of us who found, like myself, what an absolute joy it is to be able to *run* up the stairs when in a hurry—and not practically faint from shortness of breath—that is perhaps even a greater joy, the joy of living the normal kind of life everyone else seems to take for granted.

I think the first step in attacking your fat is thinking back *honestly* to when it was that you started putting weight on. If you were a kid whose mother was a force-feeder, fine. Remember that she is no longer trailing you around with a knife and fork and that you seem more than capable of getting a spoonful of sugar into your own fat face. Maybe you started getting fat when you got divorced. OK, the divorce is over, and if you want to make a new life, it's only going to be harder as a low-confidence fatty. You say your children have all left home. Well guess what. They're not coming back, so you can stop buying groceries for seven people every week. What I'm saying is that I understand as well as anyone what may have started you off on the road to Fatdom, but those are *temporary causes*, not excuses. These things happen to other people: some take to drinking, others to smoking, some to psychiatrists—and others seem to handle it themselves. There's really one trick:

> *Be aware! Be aware that fat is a result of something that gave you a loss of heart—and only overcoming and understanding that problem can make you slim again.*

I'd like to share the story of one of my Slim-U friends with you. It's about a lonely teenager named Allison who was beset by a slim family, a new town and a lack of knowledge about responsibility.

The Best Years?

When Allison first joined Slim-U, she had just entered her third year of high school. And if the last two years were any indication of things to come, the immediate future looked to be one lonely day after another. The fact that Allison was in a new town was difficult enough, but when your obesity has made you even more self-conscious, it becomes almost impossible. The fear of rejection held Allison immobile, glued to the T.V. set, living out a fantasy world. Food became her only companion. Thus the vicious cycle began, eating because we are fat and unhappy, and then becoming fatter and even more unhappy.

Now, to make matters worse, the remainder of the family was thin—and I do mean thin. Try as they might, they couldn't understand why Allison would do this to herself. Her mother pleaded with her to lose weight and sneaked around trying to catch Allison in the act. If she did, she'd yell at her, thinking that would deter her from destroying herself (our old friend shame). Dad had another idea—he'd bribe her with the promise of new clothes, or pay her compliments that were undeserved. ("Looks like you've lost a little weight—guess you've decided to stop pigging out.") Her brother Joe wasn't quite so kind—he was often the butt of the joke about his fat sister and he in turn would tease her. Each in their own way thought they had the answer. There were many nights that Allison cried herself to sleep thinking, "God, why me?" Teaching Allison to assume responsibility for her own actions was difficult. She didn't yet understand that being overweight was a choice and therefore being slim was also a choice.

I wish I could say that from the first night it was all clear sailing, but that wouldn't be the truth. Allison would leave and return to Slim-U twice within the next two years. Her high school years were less than happy, but in October of her senior year she returned and offered no excuses. Now Allison was truly ready to do battle with the fat fairy. We had a new set of phrases to discard. For example, "If I had only stuck it out I would have been slim two years ago" and "I should have stayed on the program and maybe I would have been asked to the Prom." This list went on, but you can't go forward while looking back, and we had a long way to go. So I told her no more *should have* and *could have*—let's take care of today and the hell with yesterday. With a lot of hard work, some tears and even a few angry words between us, Allison donned her cap and gown several months later 37 pounds lighter. She still had 40 pounds to lose, but she was well on her way. Allison would leave Slim-U once more, regaining eleven pounds, but now she's back to stay.

Update on Allison. Two years after graduation, she's still five pounds from her maintenance weight and it seems she just won't let that go. But remember, folks, she *has* lost 62 pounds—and *kept* it off. She has a great job and her love life has improved steadily.

So many of us, myself included, have allowed our teen years to slip by us, wishing things were different, but not willing to put forth the effort necessary to make the changes. Here's a small part of a letter Allison sent me:

> Dear B.Z.,
> I have seen people and heard of people doing marvelous things and I want to be one of them. I want moments of real happiness, though I understand there will also be sad times. B.Z., I no longer feel hopeless now that I have you in my corner. You know what I'm going through because you were also a *tubby teen*. I feel like standing on the tallest building in town and shouting "Hello, world, I'm coming back!" A better person—thinner, smarter, healthier and happier.
> Thank you so much,
> Allison

Now I don't want to hear any of you out there saying "Oh, well she's so young. It's much easier to lose weight at that age." The hell it is. Not when you don't know who you are or where your life is going. Maybe it's easier for someone with a secure home and a family who understands. The grass is always greener, friends; it's not easy for anyone to lose, but if you convince yourself that you don't have as good a chance as the guy next door, you're right—you haven't got a chance.

Control is another word we used often in this book. Certainly it is important to become aware of what it is that's making us dislike ourselves so much that we have contracted the disease of obesity (and it *is* a disease); but without using a certain amount of control on ourselves, awareness of our situation is only going to serve to make us more miserable. No one has locked us to the refrigerator and forced us to eat.

We've simply opted to be a prisoner of our own unhappiness, and we've chosen food as our refuge. We've got to learn the Art of Self-Management. If you can learn to just control yourself five minutes at a time, soon enough those five minutes add up to an hour, then a day, and before you know it a week has gone by and you've lost a couple of pounds! Just like doing paperwork in an office; you can only do one piece at a time and then attack the next job. So it is with losing weight—take it as it comes. If I had only known this on that first Longest Day of my last big diet, I would have had it a lot easier. I thought I was being practical because at 9:21 A.M. I was telling myself there were only two hours and 39 minutes until I could attack lunch! Eternity! After a time, of course, it gets easier and you find you only need the control you used to use for a minute to control yourself for an hour. And when that starts happening, gang, that's called winning.

So what we're really talking about is change. Ah, that dreaded word! The enemy of tradition! The tradition of a morning coffee cake, afternoon's hot chocolate and Oreos while watching the soaps, my traditional strawberry short-cake or lemon mousse for dessert. Again, if you say you *can't* change, you're probably right. Not until you make the choice to rid yourself of fat forever and jump off the bandwagon will you ever, ever change. You don't have to throw your whole life out of whack to go on a diet. That in itself is self-defeating. Anyone who tries to do a 360 degree turn like that is bound to turn around in a short time and say "See? I went all out, did everything I could to lose weight and it just didn't work." Of course it doesn't work, you twit. If you find yourself in the middle of a completely new lifestyle, the sheer terror of it will turn you right back to your very best and oldest friend—food. If you're used to a mid-morning snack, by all means have one. You'll find from the recipes and menu plans in this book that you really don't have to be a Joan of Arc to get through the day.

One of the keys to getting yourself in check so you can move forward and make changes is to assess exactly where you stand. That's why it truly is important to tally up the plusses in your life and take a good long look at All the Great Things about You. When you've got a good idea of all the things you've got going for yourself under your belt, it makes self-improvement a hell of a lot easier. Keep in mind that *you're the one in control,* not your husband or job or crazy children. Give them control of your feelings and you've just lost round one. Each day is for you to enjoy and share. If other people or things are involved, fine. Try to include them in your enjoyment—don't let them run it. Each day is yet another chance for making yourself, happier, better, slimmer. Speaking of the grass is always greener, let me share another eye-opening Slim-U experience.

The Slim-U Retreat

Twice a year, we at Slim-U go away with about one hundred people and spend five days eating properly, losing weight—and equally important—rapping and setting goals for ourselves. Many terrific things happen to all of us, members and directors, during these retreats.

It's seldom that a new member joins and immediately signs up for a retreat the following week. But when Ada came up to me after the meeting and said she would like to go with us and that she really needed it, I agreed. Ada was somebody I couldn't help but study from head to toe. Her lovely red hair was beautifully styled, her makeup was perfect, her clothes were straight out of *Vogue,* and other than being about 35 pounds overweight, she looked as if she didn't have a care in the world. For me, this was about to be another good lesson in how *not* to judge a book by its cover.

The day we arrived at the hotel, she looked like a model. Jewelry shone everywhere and she had more outfits with her than there were hours to wear them. The other women were turning green with envy every time she made yet another entrance in yet another set of drop-dead duds.

Each night, Ada was the first one arrive at the rap sessions and she stationed herself directly in front of where Melissa and I would stand. She never uttered a word, but she seemed intent on hanging onto every word the others had to say. We certainly don't claim to answer everyone's problems with *the* correct and only answer, but it helps everyone to know that others in the group have experienced the same rejections, hurts and depressions. On our third day there, I found an unsigned note next to my lunch plate. It read, "Tonight could we discuss how someone could *stop* wanting to die, that is to say wanting to commit suicide." I read the note several times—it isn't unusual to find a note next to my plate asking to talk about something in particular, but *suicide*? I spent a very uncomfortable afternoon wondering who was crying for help. I felt myself searching around, trying to keep tabs on everyone without anyone catching on that I was concerned.

That night Melissa and I opened the rap session by saying that one of our members was concerned about her friend who contemplates suicide from time to time, and she'd like to know how to help her. If anyone realized that the troubled party was in fact sitting in that room, they've never, to this day, mentioned it. Many suggestions were made and most of them were really good. Then, out of the blue, one of our members came up with this mind-blower.

"Many years ago, when I was young and living in Europe, I thought my life seemed hopeless and I even thought of suicide. I believed that living couldn't be more difficult, but I was wrong. Six months later I found myself in a concentration camp, and for the next few years I watched people with a great deal less to look forward to than your friend fight just to stay alive. I learned how precious this thing called life really is."

Well, talk about a show stopper. I guess it did its job, because about four months later I received this letter from Ada:

Dear B.Z.,

Did you know then or since that I am the one who had written that note about suicide? Bet not! Three years ago I had a nervous breakdown and was hospitalized for a year and two months. Since hearing Freida at that retreat I refer to that hospitalization now as my little escape from reality. God love her, she is correct—life is *so* precious and most of us never understand that until we are faced with death. I am crying so hard I can hardly see the paper, but this time it's because I'm so damn happy for a change.

I love you all,
Ada

P.S. I told Freida that very night and we spent the entire night talking and crying. Happy and on my way to being slim.

Anyone who can't learn from that is pretty far gone. *Carpe diem*, folks. Live it up every minute you can, and don't spoil those minutes with fat. Count such moments as a gift for living, not for greed and ruining the amazing thing the human body—and human life—is.

I think one of my shortcomings in all this fat business is that I forget that some people actually believe many of the fallacies around about gaining weight. Things like if you walk under a ladder you'll gain weight, or if a cookie crosses your path you'll be under the spell of fatness. And certainly no one has any hope of staying on their diet if it's Friday the thirteenth! As you know, these aren't really the kinds of things I noted earlier on in the book about lying to yourself concerning your weight. But they're just as loony as excusing big bones, thyroid problems or a sparse love life for obesity. I really do understand that one might believe some of this nonsense when they're younger, but it becomes quite obvious as the grocery bills and scales soar that water retention really isn't your problem—it's eating. You can only go on lying to yourself so long. No, wait, that isn't really true. From the looks of some people you see on the street, it seems as if they intend to lie to themselves until the day they die— which could be any minute, judging from the shape they're in. Yup, some folks will go on lying to their best friend until the day they die. Too bad they're not getting something out of it as long as they're going to all that trouble.

Don't get me wrong—I realize what's at stake here as well as you do. We could fail, right? Try to go on a diet, tell everyone all about it, and then never lose an ounce? What you're afraid of is failure, my friend. But not failure in the most important sense. We're often afraid of public failure; that is, letting down someone we love to whom we've promised we'd lose weight or failing ourselves because we absolutely told ourselves we'd be ten pounds lighter by Christmas. *Don't lose sight of your goal.* Map out your strategies beforehand with a modicum of common sense. And don't think that every time you cheat a little or glance sideways at a cupcake that all is lost. Setbacks will often happen, but they're no self-made excuse to give up all hope of ever becoming slim (although some folks will plan a cheat to disrupt a diet and tell themselves that all is lost). Dieting is as much part of the American Dream as anything. You plod along, trying to handle everything as it comes ... and if you blow it, you just pick yourself up by the bootstraps and start all over again. Because believe me, nobody else is going to pick you up. Just try to keep in mind the pro and con chart of slim vs. fat. One side is always empty, and it doesn't take an Einstein to know which one. Basically, you only fail if you choose to, and I don't known anyone who likes to fail. Remember, you're somebody special, and there will be times when everyone else will forget that. It's your job to keep it in mind—no ifs, ands or buts.

Okay, now we know that this fat didn't just hit us like a bolt out of the blue. We really worked at putting it there, bit by bit, pecan roll upon pecan roll. If you've got trouble understanding what type of situations are most dangerous to you, pretend you're a reporter. Put that press pass in your hatband and recall the five W's—who, what, where, when and why. There are people, places and things that we encounter which seem to make us more susceptible to eating than other situations. Obviously, these "W's" are to be avoided. Even if they don't make you actually overeat, sometimes they'll totally ruin your confidence in yourself— and that leads to overeating.

The Case of the Forlorn Fianceé

"If you loved me, you'd lose weight!" How many times has a fatty heard this chant? The thing the speaker doesn't realize is that no one becomes fat and uncomfortable in order to hurt or embarrass others. The person who is always hurt is the one carrying around all that excess baggage.

Take Margaret, for example. She had been dating Jim in her senior year of college, and like many other girls, was so dazzled by his straight teeth and curly hair that she failed to notice his lousy personality. Nothing ever went his way, and when things didn't turn out right it was always someone else's fault—usually Margaret's. The greatest source of his anger was the fact that Margaret was overweight. Jim took every opportunity to belittle her in front of family and friends. Of course, the more he picked at her, the more she sneaked and ate. As time went on, he became more and more abusive, calling her a "hippo" and "cow." Understandably, Margaret found herself crying constantly.

Oddly enough, for Christmas Jim presented Margaret with a small diamond ring—stating for all to hear that he only hoped it would fit her fat finger. The engagement was short-lived; on New Year's Eve he demanded the ring back and told her if she wanted to see him again, she'd better take off a ton of weight. In fact, his parting words were, "If you knock off that blubber, give me a call." Of course, besides the pain of rejection and the sting from Jim's crushing remarks, there was the embarrassment of telling people she was no longer engaged.

But behold! Margaret's sister-in-law was a member of Slim-U at the time and guessed what had really happened. She certainly understood what Margaret was going through and invited her to come to the next meeting. When I met her, all I could think of was that she looked for all the world like a little whipped puppy with all the life beat out of her. But as the weeks passed and her weight was on the way down, she seemed to be coming alive again.

One night I spoke about the way people treat you and the fact that if we allow others to hurt and embarrass us, it's really our own fault. If someone is controlling you with the promise of love or the threat of anger, it is your duty to set the rules. Nothing can exist in your life without your spoken or unspoken consent. I closed repeating what I so often say: "Remember, you are somebody special, and if people sometimes forget, it's up to you to remind them."

Meanwhile, rumors had come back to Margaret that not only had Jim been dating someone else, but he was still making fun of her from a distance. Margaret was losing weight so quickly that I was amazed at the difference from week to week. Soon, as is the way with all rumors, word began to get back to Jim about how great Margaret looked and how happy and carefree she seemed to be. And then, Margaret arrived home from work one night and there was Jim, sitting in his car in her driveway. For one fleeting moment she felt a sense of panic, but Margaret drew herself up and walked over to his car. He looked her up and down and then said *now* he'd like to start dating her again—but she'd better not get fat. I love this letter with Margaret's reply—bet you will, too!

Dear B.Z.,

I never thought I could do it, but I did. I said, "Gee, Jim, thanks for the wonderful offer. But if you were the last man on earth, I'd become a nun." As I turned and walked in the house I felt so proud. Jim was right—I did need to lose weight, but what I didn't need was him. It's been a year today, B.Z., and I am still slim, and where's Jim? Who the hell cares?

Your skinny Minnie,
Margaret

Strength builds strength and weakness builds weakness. Hooray for Margaret and hooray for all of us every time we spy a trouble spot coming and manage to avoid it!

There's no simple way to *avoid* overeating, though. It's not as though you can take a detour and go around it. And it doesn't just happen; you've got to work at it. If your hobby happens to be sitting around staring at the refrigerator deciding on new, fun ways to decorate it, I suggest another pastime. Keeping yourself busy—your hands especially—is the key to remaining faithful to your diet. Start on that project you've been putting off for so long. You'll be surprised how much extra time you have now that you're not locking yourself in the kitchen all day. And you'll discover that there are many ways to treat yourself besides rewarding yourself with food at every turn. That is the most negative form of reinforcement and I assure you that you'll be delighted when you find out how many other nice things there are in the world you can treat yourself to—and they satisfy so much longer!

Now, I realize that it would take a superhuman person to be on a diet and *never* cheat. But the most dangerous thing that can happen is to cheat and then punish yourself for it. To make yourself feel miserable for an extended period because you gave in to a bowl of ice cream is self-defeating and leads to a level of frustration that is commonly followed by binging. Once you begin to punish yourself for small failures, you very often bring yourself back to square one—with a spurt of binging along the way. Guilt and frustration simply have no benefits. You waver for a minute, fine. Put on the blinders, get up and keep going. Nothing will make you feel better than knowing that you have the control to get back on the track. Same thing applies when you reach a plateau where you remain at a constant weight for a while. This is why we weigh-in only once a week according to Slim-U rules. It's pretty discouraging to truly work at your diet and stay at the same weight for a week or two. Try to get on the scales only once a week (it's really much more rewarding). A plateau of weight constancy never lasts more than two weeks—if you're really staying on your diet. And always keep in mind the true meaning of the word plateau: it's a level place to kind of take a breather before you start climbing to your next peak.

Professionally Speaking

Over the years, I've learned never to think of my Slim-U members as a group of people, but rather as individual people sitting in a group. There are as many unique stories as there are people filling the room—and this incident taught me that you sure can't tell the Chiefs from the Indians without a score card.

Terry had been a member for about eight weeks, and one thing I remembered most about her was that she stayed at the end of the sessions to talk to me. In fact, she seemed to have more than the usual amount of questions. I gathered from the information she fed me that she had begun gaining weight about seven years prior to starting at Slim-U and expressed that fact that she was at a loss to find the reason for her steady weight gains—she was happily married, had two children, a career and was very attractive. The only thing I could put my finger on during our conversations was the fact that she seemed to lack confidence. She constantly asked me

"I'm not bothering you, am I?" or "Am I asking too many questions?" I finally brought it to her attention and she replied, "I guess I sometimes do question my abilities. Even when I know I can do something, I'm afraid to try."

She never missed a meeting, though, and she'd often nod her head in agreement while I delivered my talk. One evening as she turned around and left the scales, I saw two of my new members looking as if they'd just seen the Ghost of the Chocolate Mousse. After much whispering, they decided they could contain themselves no longer and they took me aside.

"Excuse me, is Terry a member of this group?" Elaine asked.

"Sure is," I said. "I noticed a surprised look on your face when you first saw her. Mind if I ask why?"

"Well", Elaine said, "she's our therapist—and we didn't know she came here."

Well, if I thought they looked shocked, I truly took the cake (you should excuse the expression). For a moment I thought "Good grief! How can I get up here now in front of a pro? Anything I say will sound dumb. Why is she here in *my* diet group?" After a minute or so of panic, I walked to the front of the room and could tell by the look on her face that she knew the cat was out of the bag. During the next week I received this letter.

Dear B.Z.,

Shame on me for not telling you, and shame on you for thinking it would make a difference. During the past weeks I've been sitting and listening to your weekly talks. I've been taking from you and returning little or nothing. My training is in the field of psychology, so if anyone should be able to psych themselves into not eating, it should be me. Wrong. Someone once said, "A little learning is a dangerous thing." This applies in my case—I know the proper responses, defense mechanisms, alternate behavior patterns and the other tricks of the "behavior modification trade." None of them has helped me as much as you have. I can't tell you how thrilled I am having lost 27 pounds in the last weeks. Slim-U gives me something I haven't been able to give myself—confidence and love. Nowhere is it written that a "helper never needs help." Thanks for helping me.

Terry

See what I mean? No one has an easier time of it than anyone else. One would think that dieting would be a cinch for Terry, but lo and behold, she turned out to be human, too. Even with an occupation that depended on her helping people control their own lives day in and day out, Terry took a while before she concentrated on #1 and decided to become her own best friend. Like I say, no one has a patent on self-control. Terry was so busy rescuing everyone else that she avoided facing herself. We all must do what she did—wake up and explore our past mistakes. Not to explore them for the sake of punishing ourselves for all the months or years we were self-abusive, but to realize when and where we went wrong so we can sidestep those pitfalls when we see them coming next time. Success is no mistake, my friends, and it sure takes some work. But I swear to you—stick with me and work at leaving your fat behind, and I promise you that someday, someday *soon*, you too can be convinced that the zipper was not invented as a form of medieval torture.

I love you all for trying and I know you can do it. Go to it, folks—it won't be long before you too can say "It's all behind me now!"

Appendix

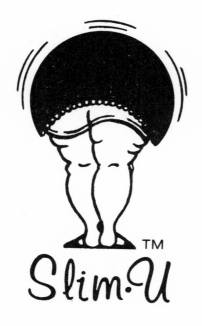

Slim·U

It's always helpful to have some guidelines. Here are some hints I give to the Slim-U groups—which food falls into which group (there is no chocolate group, so look no further) and some things that are definitely *off* the list for all of us who are serious about losing weight and keeping it off!

You'll also find lots of really tasty recipes—I assure you they're tastier than the paper they're written on. They're a conglomeration of some of my own and many our Slim-U friends have given us over the years—I promise you you'll find some mouth-watering ones!

Enjoy!

The Slim-U Plan

Equivalent Value Chart

This program has proven to be a successful plan for hundreds of men and women. If you do not deviate (take away or add to) from the prescribed program, you will surely reduce your weight, look better, feel better and at the same time adjust your appetite to retain the weight loss. This **WAY OF LIFE** will then become a simple procedure and just as you always reached for the wrong food, you will now think only in terms of your proper eating habits.

1. Eat only food listed in the menu plan in quantities specified.

NEVER SKIP A MEAL!
DO NOT COUNT CALORIES
WEIGH AND MEASURE ALL FOODS

2. Use as desired the following items.

Bouillon
Carbonated beverages
    (noncaloric)
Clear soup (fat free)
Herbs
Horseradish
Lemon–lime
Mustard

Salt, pepper
Seltzer
Tea–coffee
Tomato juice
Vinegar, spices
Water
Worcestershire sauce

Vegetables

3. Eat all you want of the following, raw or cooked, without fat or sauces or salad oil dressing, either at meals or between meals if you have a feeling of hunger.

Asparagus
(Natural diuretic)
Beet greens
Broccoli
Cabbage
Cauliflower
Celery
Chinese cabbage
Cucumber
Endive
Escarole
Green and red pepper
Lettuce

Mung bean sprouts
Mushrooms
Mustard greens
Parsley
Dill pickles
Pimentos
Radishes
Sauerkraut (own juice)
Spinach
Squash, summer
String beans
Watercress

Limited as Directed

4. Eat the following as indicated on your menu plan. Vary your selection from day to day (4 oz. serving). Eat a dark

green or yellow vegetable each day. (*) These vegetables can be eliminated entirely.

Artichokes	Oyster plant
Bamboo shoots	Parsnips
Beets	Peas
Brussel sprouts	Pumpkin
Carrots*	Scallions
Eggplant	Squash
Green beans (mature)	Tomato*
Okra	Turnips
Onions*	

Fruits

5. Eat three fruits a day—one of which should be a vitamin C fruit. Men are allowed five fruits a day. You may eat any fruit in season except: bananas, cherries, watermelon, dried fruits, grapes, papayas, mangos, avocados.

Fruit equivalents (no sugar added): The following equal one (1) fruit:

4 oz. unsweetened fruit juice	½ cup pineapple (in its own juice)
½ cantaloupe	½ grapefruit
¼ honeydew melon	½ cup fruit cocktail
½ cup berries	

Proteins

6. Proteins consist of eggs, hard cheese (2 oz. daily limit), cottage cheese, pot cheese or farmer cheese, lean meats, fish and poultry. Broil, pan broil, bake or roast meat, fish or poultry—DO NOT FRY. Remove all visible fat before eating— DO NOT EAT GRAVIES OR SAUCES. Chicken and quail may be substituted for fish. Eggs are limited to 4–7 per week. Cook eggs in shell or poach or scramble (without fat—use Pam). If using an egg substitute—4 a week limit.

First Choice

Abalone	Kidney
Bass	Lobster
Brains	Lungs
Chicken, breast	Mussels
Cod	Oysters
Finnan Haddie	Pike
Flounder	Scallops
Haddock	Shrimp
Halibut	Sturgeon—fresh
Heart—beef	Trout—brook

Second Choice

Bluefish	Shad
Bonito	Shad roe
Butterfish	Trout—lake
Chicken	Tuna fish (fresh or canned,
Eels	water packed)
Kidney—beef	Turkey, light meat only
Liver	Veal
Mackerel	White fish
Pheasant	(8 oz. raw fillet, 6 oz.
Rabbit	cooked per portion)
Salmon (canned)	(10 oz. raw with skin and
Swordfish	bone)

3 Times Weekly

Beef	Salmon, fresh
Frankfurter (8 oz.)	Turkey, dark meat (no skin)
Lamb	

NO COLD CUTS

7. Eat enriched white or 100% whole wheat bread. Two 1-oz. slices is your daily limit or four slices of very thinly sliced bread. *Cold* cereals may be eaten for breakfast *with a protein*

if bread is omitted. The *only* cereals allowed are of the high-protein type. ½ cup cereal equals 1 slice of bread.

8. Your diet includes two 8 oz. cups of skim or fat-free milk. You may use some of this in your beverage or you may drink it at mealtime or in-between meals. Fat-free buttermilk or evaporated skim milk may be substituted. Diet ice cream equals 1 noncitrus fruit and 1 milk. Men are allowed 4 cups of milk a day.

Daily Requirements

> 3 fruits—one of which should be a vitamin C fruit
> 2 (8-oz.) glasses of skim milk
> 12 oz. of protein—meat, fish or poultry
> > 2 oz. for breakfast or 1 egg or ¼ cup cottage cheese or pot cheese
> > 4 oz. for lunch or ⅔ cup cottage cheese or pot cheese or 2 oz. of hard cheese or 2 eggs
> > 6 oz. for dinner
> Free *Number 3* vegetables

Daily Options

> 4 oz. *Number 4* vegetables
> 1 tablespoon diet margarine or diet mayonnaise or vegetable oil
> 1 tablespoon diet salad dressing
> 2 oz. white enriched bread or whole wheat bread or ½ cup cereal for breakfast

Slim-U Recipes

Breakfast Sandwich
Serves 4
1 serving = 1 bread, 2 oz. protein, ½ fruit

4 slices bread, toasted
1 (8-oz.) can sliced pineapple in own juice, drained
1⅓ cups cottage cheese
cinnamon

Spread cottage cheese on toast. Top with pineapple slice and sprinkle with cinnamon. Broil 6 inches from heat for 4 to 5 minutes.

Complete Breakfast
Serves 1
1 serving = 2 oz. protein, 4 oz. *number 4* vegetable, 1 bread

> 1 egg
> 1 slice very thin bread
> 1 small tomato
> salt and pepper

Scoop out pulp of tomato. Break egg into tomato and sprinkle with salt and pepper. Bake at 350° for 15 minutes until egg is set. Place on toasted bread.

Apple Muffins
Serves 6
1 serving = ½ fruit, ½ bread, 1 oz. protein

> 3 apples, sliced (you may use blueberries, strawber-
> ries, peaches)
> 3 slices white bread
> 3 eggs
> 1½ pkgs. Sweet 'N Low
> ½ t. vanilla extract
> 1 t. coconut extract

Put eggs, Sweet 'N Low and extracts in a bowl. Beat with a mixer. Then add apples and bread (tear bread into cubes), stir with a spoon. Spray muffin tin with Pam, bake at 350° for 45 minutes.

Apple Tidbits
Serves 5
1 serving = 1 fruit

> ½ cup water
> ½ cup unsweetened apple juice concentrate
> 4 whole cloves

¼ t. ginger
¼ t. cinnamon
4 apples, cored, sliced and diced

In a saucepan combine first 4 ingredients. Bring to a boil and add apples. Cook till tender. Sprinkle with cinnamon.

Omelet
Serves 4
1 serving = 2 oz. protein, ½ bread

4 eggs separated
salt and pepper to taste
2 T. water
2 oz. bread broken into pieces

Beat whites with salt until stiff. Beat yolk with pepper, water and bread till fluffy. Fold whites into yolks. Spray pan with Pam. Pour eggs into heated skillet. Cover and reduce to low. Cook 8 to 10 minutes.

Sunny-Side-Up Eggs and Muffins
Serves 4
1 serving = 2 oz. protein, 1 bread all

2 bagels, split and toasted
4 t. prepared mustard
tarragon
4 eggs
salt and pepper to taste

Spread bagel with mustard and sprinkle with tarragon. Place in a 9-inch skillet with ovenproof handle or in layer cake pan sprayed with nonstick coating. Break an egg over each bagel half. Sprinkle with salt and pepper. Broil about 6 inches from heat source 4 to 5 minutes or until eggs are set. If desired, garnish with parsley.

Apple Butter
½ cup = 1 fruit

1 pkg. unsweetened strawberry flavored instant drink mix
2 pkgs. Sweet 'N Low
3 cups diet applesauce
1 stick cinnamon

Mix ingredients in a saucepan and cook slowly about 15 minutes or until mixture becomes thick. Place in container and refrigerate.

Apple Crumb Special
Serves 4
1 serving = 2 oz. protein, ½ fruit, ½ bread

6 oz. cottage cheese
2 eggs, beaten
1 large apple sliced
4 slices thin bread, crumbed
1 t. vanilla
1 pkg. Sweet 'N Low
⅛ t. buttered salt
1 T. lemon juice

Mix all ingredients in casserole. Sprinkle with cinnamon and bake at 375° for 30 minutes.

Pancakes
Serves 1
1 serving = 2 oz. protein, 1 slice bread, ¼ fruit

2 oz. cottage cheese
1 slice bread
¼ sliced apple, blueberries, strawberries, etc.
cinnamon
Sweet 'N Low

Blend in blender cottage cheese, bread and dash of water to start blender. Pour into a *hot* skillet until brown on bottom. Add apple slices to top and broil 4 inches from broiler until fruit is cooked and top browned. Sprinkle with cinnamon and Sweet 'N Low.

Jelly Roll
Serves 2
1 serving = 2 oz. protein, 1 milk

2 eggs separated
1 t. vanilla
¼ t. salt
½ t. baking soda
1 T. water
¾ cup dry milk
¾ t. cream of tartar
5 pkgs. Sweet 'N Low

In bowl combine egg yolks, water and vanilla, then add milk and mix till smooth. Beat egg whites until foamy, then add salt, cream of tartar, baking soda and Sweet 'N Low until stiff. Fold egg whites into milk mixture. Spread in a 9 × 11-inch pan. Bake at 350° for 8 minutes. Remove and roll up with a sheet of wax paper to cool. When cool, unroll, remove wax paper, spread with diet jelly and reroll. Slice to serve.

Marge Regan's Pineapple Bread Pudding
Serves 2
1 serving = 4 oz. protein, 1 slice bread, 1 fruit, ½ cup milk

2 slices white bread
1 cup liquid skim milk
3 pkgs. Sweet 'N Low
6 oz. cottage cheese
2 eggs
½ t. vanilla
pinch of salt
cinnamon
1 cup crushed pineapple (drained)

Spray 8-inch pan with Pam. Toast and cube bread, place in bottom of pan. Mix cottage cheese and pineapple together with fork until blended. Spread mixture over bread cubes. Mix with electric mixer, your eggs, Sweet 'N Low skim milk and extract. Pour over cheese mixture and sprinkle with cinnamon. Bake at 350° for 45 minutes.

Cantaloupe Ideal
Serves 1
1 serving = 1 fruit, 2 oz. protein

½ cantaloupe
2 oz. ricotta cheese
1 pkg. Sweet 'N Low
½ t. vanilla

Mix ricotta cheese, Sweet 'N Low, and vanilla together and scoop into center of cantaloupe.

Broccoli Spread
Serves 2
1 serving = 2 oz. protein, ⅛ cup diet mayonnaise

1 (10 oz.) package frozen chopped broccoli
2 large eggs, hard cooked
¼ cup diet mayonnaise
1 T. prepared mustard
1 T. fresh lemon juice
3 T. grated parmesan cheese
salt and pepper to taste, if desired

Cook broccoli according to package directions. Turn into a strainer and drain out all liquid. Chop very fine. Chop eggs and add to broccoli and remaining ingredients. Mix well and allow to chill to blend all flavors. Serve as a spread or a dip for assorted raw vegetables.

Garden Salad
Serves 4
1 serving = 1 tablespoon oil

⅓ cup oil
3 T. red-wine vinegar
2 T. minced red or green onion
½ t. each salt and Sweet 'N Low
1 cucumber, peeled, split, seeded (optional) and cut
    in ¼-inch strips
½ cup radishes
3 to 4 cups torn lettuce or escarole
fresh-ground pepper to taste

In salad bowl mix oil, vinegar, onion, salt and Sweet 'N Low. Add cucumber, green pepper and radishes, toss to mix. Just before serving, add lettuce and toss.

Spinach Salad
Serves 2
1 serving = 2 oz. protein, 1 oz. *number 4* vegetable

        1 lb. fresh spinach
        4 hard boiled eggs, chopped
        imitation bacon bits
        ¼ onion chopped
        2 T. diet italian dressing
        salt to taste

Tear spinach leaves in small pieces. Combine with eggs and imitation bacon bits, add onions. Toss lightly. Add dressing and salt. Serve immediately.

Shrimp and Pea Salad
Serves 2
1 serving = 4 oz. protein, 4 oz. *number 4* vegetable

        1 cup shrimp
        1 cup cooked peas
        ¼ cup diet mayonnaise
        1 pkg. lime flavored gelatin
        salt and pepper to taste
        2 green peppers
        lettuce

Mix ¼ cup diet mayonnaise with shrimp and peas, season with salt and pepper. Dissolve gelatin in 1 cup boiling water and add 1 cup ice water. Add shrimp and pea mixture. Cut off tops of green peppers and remove seeds. Pour gelatin mixture into pepper cups and chill. Serve on lettuce and top with a dash of mayonnaise.

Cucumber and Onion Salad
Serves 2
1 serving = 4 oz. *number 4* vegetable

4 cucumbers, peeled and thinly sliced
1 t. salt
1 cup Japanese seasoned rice wine vinegar or white
    wine vinegar
1 pkg. Sweet 'N Low
2 green onions, thinly sliced
salt and pepper to taste

Sprinkle cucumbers with salt; let stand 15 minutes; drain. Combine cucumbers with remaining ingredients; marinate in refrigerator for at least 1 hour. Serve chilled.

Cucumber Salad
Serves 1
1 serving = 1 oz. *number 4* vegetable

4 cucumbers, thinly sliced
½ onion, sliced
¼ cup water
¼ cup vinegar
½ pkg. Sweet 'N Low
1 t. minced garlic
salt and pepper to taste

Combine all ingredients, cover bowl, refrigerate at least one hour.

Cucumber Salad
Unlimited

4 cucumbers, sliced thin
1 onion, chopped
½ pkg. Sweet 'N Low
dash pepper
½ cup vinegar
1 T. lemon juice

Mix all ingredients in bowl and refrigerate overnight.

Cole Slaw
Serves 4

1 serving = 2 oz. *number 4* vegetable, 1 tablespoon milk, ¼ tablespoon diet mayonnaise, ¼ teaspoon diet salad dressing

½ head cabbage
½ green pepper
¼ cucumber (with skin)
½ carrot
4 radishes
1 T. vinegar
¼ cup skim milk
1 T. diet mayonnaise
1 t. low-calorie thousand island dressing
½ pkg. Sweet 'N Low

Shred all vegetables. In a small cup mix last 5 ingredients. Season to taste. Combine vegetables and dressing. Refrigerate.

Summer Salad
Serves 2
1 serving = 4 oz. *number 4* vegetable

2 large tomatoes
1 small onion (preferably red)
½ t. salt
1 T. oil
1 T. red wine vinegar

Seed and slice pepper. Slice tomatoes and onions thinly. Place all ingredients in a covered bowl. Mix. Chill for 30 minutes (24 hours is better).

Bean and Beef Salad
Serves 1
1 serving = 4 oz. *number 4* vegetable, 4 oz. protein, 1 tablespoon oil

1 T. prepared mustard
2 T. vinegar
¼ cup oil
basil
salt
pepper
1 can (15 to 16 oz.) whole or uncut green beans, well
    drained
1 small onion, sliced thin
1½ cups julienne-cut cooked lean steak or roast (8
    oz.)
greens
sliced tomatoes

In bowl beat mustard, vinegar, oil, ½ teaspoon each basil and salt and ¼ teaspoon pepper until blended. Toss in beans, onion and beef; marinate at room temperature at least 30 minutes. Serve on greens with tomatoes seasoned with basil, salt and pepper to taste.

Salad
Unlimited

2 T. water
2 T. cider vinegar
2 T. vegetable oil
1 pkg. Sweet 'N Low
½ t. salt
1 cup thinly sliced radishes
1 cup thinly sliced celery

Mix water, vinegar, oil, sweetener and salt. Add radishes and celery. Toss. Cover and chill 10–15 minutes.

Chinese Vegetable Salad
Serves 4
1 serving = 1 tablespoon mayonnaise

½ cup canned chinese vegetables, drained and rinsed
¼ cup bean sprouts
¼ cup diet mayonnaise
1 T. onion, chopped
1 small clove garlic

Combine all ingredients, marinate 4 hours. Serve on a lettuce leaf.

Broccoli–Cheese Dish
Serves 6
1 serving = 4 oz. protein, 4 oz. *number 4* vegetable

    2 cups cottage cheese
    ⅓ cup grated parmesan cheese
    2 pkgs frozen chopped broccoli thawed (10 oz. each)
    2 cups Slim-U tomato sauce

To make Slim-U tomato sauce take 1 large can tomato juice, 1 teaspoon each of garlic, oregano, parsley, basil and 1 bay leaf. Place all ingredients in saucepan and simmer until thickened.

Place broccoli in a $12 \times 8 \times 2$-inch pan sprayed with Pam. Pour half the sauce over broccoli and then spoon on cottage cheese. Pour on remaining sauce and sprinkle on parmesan cheese. Bake at 350° for 25 to 30 minutes.

Stuffed Tomatoes
Serves 8
1 serving = 4 oz. *number 4* vegetable, 1 bread allowance

    8 small tomatoes
    Pam
    4 cups zucchini, chopped
    2 cups mushrooms, sliced
    1 medium onion, chopped
    1 clove garlic, minced
    1 t. dried basil
    Sweet 'N Low equivalent to ½ t. sugar
    1 cup plain croutons

Cut tops off tomatoes, scoop out and reserve pulp. Sprinkle shells with salt. Chop pulp. Spray saucepan with Pam and cook: pulp, zucchini, mushrooms, onion, garlic, 1 t. salt, basil, Sweet 'N Low and dash of pepper over medium high heat for about 20 minutes or until liquid evaporates. Stir in croutons and spoon mix into shells. Place shells in baking dish and bake covered at 350° for 15 minutes. Uncover and bake an additional 10 minutes.

Asparagus Vinaigrette
Serves 1
1 serving = 1 tablespoon oil

1 lb. asparagus
Salt and pepper to taste
1 packet or cube instant chicken broth
1 T. wine vinegar
1 T. salad oil
1 scallion, peeled and finely minced

Break asparagus near bottom of stems—they will snap at the tender point (peel stem ends if desired and serve raw or add to soup). Wash asparagus thoroughly; tie in a bundle and stand upright in a tall pot or coffee pot. Steam just until tender and still bright green, about 8 minutes. Remove asparagus to serving plate; discard tie. To ¾ cup of the cooking liquid, add instant chicken broth, wine vinegar (or lemon juice), oil, scallion, salt and pepper. Pour over asparagus, serve warm or cool.

Mushrooms Vinaigrette
Serves 1
1 serving = 1 tablespoon oil

1 lb. mushrooms
Salt and pepper to taste
1 packet or cube instant chicken broth
1 T. wine vinegar

1 T. salad oil
1 scallion, peeled and finely minced

Buy 1 pound large white mushrooms, looking for caps with closed bottoms for freshness. Cut off bottoms of stems; wipe caps with damp towel to clean (if immersed in water, mushrooms lose flavor; no need to peel unless mushrooms are nicked or spotted). Slice lengthwise. Heat 1 tablespoon oil in pan, add mushrooms, toss over briefly, just until golden. Bring ¾ cup water to boil. Add instant chicken broth, vinegar, oil, scallion, salt and pepper. Pour sauce over mushrooms.

Vinaigrette Dressing
Unlimited

½ cup white wine vinegar
¼ cup water
½ t. mustard
½ t. basil
½ t. celery salt
½ t. oregano
½ t. onion flakes
4 pkgs. Sweet 'N Low
dash pepper

Mix all ingredients in container and shake. Keep refrigerated.

Veggie Potpourri
Serves 4
1 serving = 2 oz. *number 4* vegetable, 1½ teaspoons of oil

1½ cups finely cut up cabbage
1 cup grated carrots (one carrot)
½ cup finely chopped onion

½ cup chopped celery
¾ t. salt
2 T. oil
½ cup boiling water

Combine all ingredients and cook till tender. Approximately 20 minutes.

Carrots Supreme
Serves 5
1 serving = 4 oz. *number 4* vegetable

16 oz. carrots
1 t. instant beef bouillon
1 cup hot water
1 small chopped onion
1 t. worcestershire sauce

Add all ingredients to baking dish and bake at 325° until tender. About 30 minutes.

Cheese and Spinach Casserole
Serves 1
1 serving = 4 oz. protein, ¼ milk

1 pkg. chopped spinach
1 egg, hard boiled
1 oz. grated cheese
1 t. onion, chopped
¼ cup dry skim milk
⅛ t. nutmeg

Cook spinach by package directions. Drain. Add onion, milk, nutmeg, egg, salt and pepper to taste. Put in small baking dish and sprinkle with cheese. Bake at 375° for 20 minutes.

Green Bean Chili
Serves 4
1 serving = 6 oz. protein, 4 oz. *number 4* vegetable

1½ lbs. lean ground beef or veal
1 large red onion, chopped (1⅓ cups)
2 small green peppers, chopped (1 cup)
2 lb. size french style green beans, drained
1 (18 oz.) can tomato juice
1 t. garlic
1 t. ground cumin
½ t. salt
¼ t. pepper
3 T. chili powder
2 pkgs. Sweet 'N Low

Brown ground beef or veal. Drain well. Add remaining ingredients stirring frequently. Cook uncovered for 30 minutes.

Broccoli Souffle
Serves 4
1 serving = ⅛ cup skim milk

2 cups cooked broccoli, drained and finely chopped
¼ t. nutmeg
salt and pepper to taste
¼ cup evaporated skim milk

Season broccoli with nutmeg, salt and pepper. Fold in milk; place in 1 quart casserole. Bake at 400° for about 20 minutes.

Great Zucchini
Unlimited

5 medium zucchini
½ t. salt
1 t. salad herbs
½ cup water

Slice zucchini. Combine all ingredients in a medium frying pan. Cover and cook about 10–12 minutes.

Herbed Green Peas
Serves 5
1 serving = 4 oz. *number 4* vegetable

2 (10 oz.) pkgs. frozen peas, unthawed
½ t. salt
dash ground pepper
¼ t. basil
¼ cup water

Place all ingredients in sauce pan and cook for the time recommended on vegetable package.

Broccoli and Chestnuts
Serves 4
1 serving = 4 oz. *number 4* vegetables

1 pkg. frozen broccoli
2 cans water chestnuts, thinly sliced

4 T. soy sauce
Sweet 'N Low to taste

Thaw broccoli and mix with remaining ingredients. Toss.

Baked Squash
Serves 1
1 serving = 4 oz. *number 4* vegetable, ½ teaspoon margarine

1 (4 oz.) acorn squash
½ t. diet margarine
salt and pepper

Cut squash in half. Remove seeds. Brush lightly with melted margarine, sprinkle with salt and pepper. Bake in dish, cut side down, 20 minutes. Turn and bake 40 minutes longer.

Braised Escarole and Tomatoes
Serves 2
1 serving = 4 oz. *number 4* vegetable

1 medium clove garlic, crushed
dash oil
1 can (8 oz.) tomatoes, cut up
1 head escarole, rinsed well and drained

In medium skillet, saute garlic in hot oil until lightly browned. Add tomatoes, then as much escarole as will fit in skillet. Cover and steam 10 to 12 minutes, stirring occasionally and adding more escarole as it cooks down.

Italian Scallops
Serves 4
1 serving = 6 oz. protein, 4 oz. *number 4* vegetable

    1½ lbs. scallops
    1 green pepper, diced
    ½ cup mushrooms, sliced
    ¼ cup lemon juice
    1½ cups tomato juice
    ¾ t. garlic powder
    ½ t. onion salt
    1 T. wine vinegar
    ½ t. basil
    1 t. diced onion

In small saucepan, mix tomato juice, garlic powder, onion salt, basil, vinegar and diced onion. Cook over medium heat 15 minutes or until sauce begins to thicken. Add peppers and mushrooms. Cook an additional 10 minutes. Place scallops in baking dish. Pour lemon juice over scallops. Bake at 350° for 12 minutes. Drain off juice. Add tomato sauce mixture and bake at 400° for 10 minutes.

Shrimp Scampi
Serves 2
1 serving = 6 oz. protein, 2 oz. *number 4* vegetable

    ¼ cup chicken stock or water
    ½ large onion or 6 shallots
    1 large clove garlic, minced
    2 t. minced parsley
    dash oregano
    1 lb. prawn or colossal shrimp, cleaned

In heavy saucepan holding stock or water, steam all ingredients except shrimp for 10 minutes. Bake shrimp in 350°

oven for 25 minutes. Add sauce and brown in broiler for 5 minutes.

Chinese Shrimp
Serves 4
1 serving = 4 oz. protein, 2 oz. _number 4_ vegetable

    1 lb. uncooked shrimp, shelled and deveined
    1 lb. bean sprouts
    1 clove garlic
    2 t. ginger
    1 onion, sliced
    1 green pepper, sliced
    2 stalks celery, sliced
    1 small can mushrooms
    2 chicken bouillon cubes
    2 cups water
    4 T. soy sauce
    1 T. chives

Drain bean sprouts and wash. Put all ingredients in a saucepan, cover and cook for 20 minutes.

Tuna Casserole
Serves 1
1 serving = 6 oz. protein

    1 can tuna packed in water
    1 can bean sprouts
    1 cup mushrooms, sliced
    1 cup celery, chopped
    ½ cup tomato juice
    1 t. onion flakes
    ¼ t. ginger
    dash pepper
    3 T. soy sauce

Combine all ingredients except tuna and sprouts in pan and cook 5 minutes. Add sprouts and cook another 5 minutes. Stir in tuna and pour into casserole dish. Bake at 350° for 20 minutes.

Tuna Casserole
Serves 1
1 serving = 6 oz. protein, 4 oz. tomato juice

½ cup tomato juice
1 t. onion, chopped
¼ t. ginger
1 cup sliced mushrooms
3 T. soy sauce
dash pepper
1 lb. can bean sprouts
6 oz. canned tuna in water

Combine first 7 ingredients in pan and cook 5 minutes. Add sprouts and cook 5 more minutes. Stir in tuna. Bake in a 1 quart dish at 350° for 20 minutes.

Scallop Sticks
Serves 2
1 serving = 6 oz. protein, 1 fruit

1 lb. scallops
4 oz. button mushrooms
1 can pineapple chunks, drained
green pepper, cut in 1-inch pieces
¼ cup each:
    parsley, chopped
    soy sauce
    lemon juice
dash pepper

Combine all ingredients in bowl and marinate 30 minutes, stirring occasionally. Alternate peppers, mushrooms, pineapple, and scallops. Broil lightly until browned.

Easy Chicken Creole
Serves 2
1 serving = 6 oz. protein, 2 oz. *number 4* vegetable

    1 large onion, chopped
    ¾ cup diced or chopped frozen or fresh green
        pepper
    1 large clove garlic, crushed
    1 cup Slim-U tomato sauce (page 149)
    2¼ cups chicken broth
    ½ t. salt
    ¼ t. Sweet 'N Low
    ¼ t. hot-pepper sauce
    2 cups cubed chicken
    fresh-ground pepper to taste

In large skillet, saute onion, green peppers, and garlic until tender, stirring occasionally. Stir in tomato sauce, broth, salt, Sweet 'N Low, and pepper sauce. Cook and stir until mixture comes to a boil and thickens. Simmer uncovered for 5 minutes, stirring occasionally. Stir in chicken and season with fresh-ground pepper. Heat until hot.

Mushroom Stuffed Chicken
Serves 1
1 serving = 5 oz. cooked protein, ½ oz. cheese protein

    ¼ cup fresh mushrooms, chopped
    ½ t. liquid chicken base
    ½ oz. Neufchatel cheese
    2 (4 oz.) chicken breasts, boned
    ½ cup white wine

Slightly flatten chicken breasts. Stuff each with half of stuffing mix. Roll, place in a shallow baking dish. Pour wine over chicken. Sprinkle with paprika. Cover and bake at 350° for 40 minutes. Pour juice over chicken when served.

Japanese Chicken
Serves 2
1 serving = 6 oz. protein

4 chicken breasts
⅓ cup wine vinegar
½ cup soy sauce
1 clove garlic, minced
1 pkg. Sweet 'N Low
¼ t. ground ginger

Mix all ingredients and marinate chicken 1 or 2 hours. Bake chicken in shallow pan at 325° for 1 hour. Baste with marinade often.

Chicken and Broccoli
Serves 2
1 serving = 6 oz. protein

Chicken:
    1 egg white
    1 t. minced, peeled fresh gingerroot or ¼ t.
        ground ginger
    1 lb. boneless, skinless chicken breast cut across
        grain into ¼ inch wide strips

Sauce:
    ¼ cup soy sauce
    ¼ cup chicken broth
    2 T. minced, peeled fresh gingerroot or ½ t.
        ground ginger
    1 t. vegetable oil

To Finish
    4 T. vegetable oil
    4 cups broccoli florets
    ¼ cup sliced green onions or scallions

Chicken: Mix egg white, soy sauce, and fresh ginger in a bowl. Add chicken and stir to coat thoroughly.

Sauce: Mix all ingredients in a small bowl

To Finish: In a wok or large skillet heat 2 tablespoons of the oil over high heat. Add broccoli and stir briskly for 1–2 minutes, until crisp-tender. Transfer to a large bowl. Add remaining 2 tablespoons of oil to skillet and heat over moderately high heat. Add chicken and cook 4–5 minutes, stirring constantly, until pieces separate and turn white. Return broccoli to skillet; add sauce mixture. Stir briskly for 20–30 seconds, until chicken is glazed. Sprinkle with green onions and serve.

Hurry-Up Chicken
Serves 2
1 serving = 6 oz. protein

4 chicken breasts
3 t. chicken bouillon
½ cup water
½ t. diet Italian dressing
¼ onion, chopped
¼ celery, chopped

In pan place onions, celery, broth, water and dressing. Simmer until vegetables are tender. Add chicken and more water if needed. Simmer covered for 30 minutes.

Orange Chicken Salad
Serves 1
1 serving = 4 oz. protein, 1 fruit, ½ teaspoon diet mayonnaise

    1 eating orange
    4 oz. cooked chicken, white meat
    ¼ cup celery, chopped
    1 t. diet mayonnaise
    ¼ cup chopped orange pulp

Cut orange in half. Remove pulp. Combine chicken, pulp, celery, and mayonnaise. Fill orange halves, and arrange on a bed of lettuce.

Enchilada
Serves 1
1 serving = 4 oz. protein, 1 slice bread, 4 oz. *number 4* vegetable

    ½ cup diet catsup
    1 T. dehydrated onion flakes
    1 medium tomato, chopped
    ½ clove garlic, minced
    1 T. chopped green chili peppers
    dash Sweet 'N Low
    ½ t. ground cumin
    ¼ t. salt
    ¼ t. oregano
    ¼ t. basil
    2 oz. monterey jack cheese, shredded
    1 slice bread, toasted

Put all ingredients (except cheese and toast) in saucepan and simmer 15 minutes. Dip toast into mixture and moisten both sides. Put coated toast in small oven-proof baking dish and top with cheese and remaining sauce. Bake at 350° for 15–20 minutes.

Quick Lunch
Serves 1
1 serving = 4 oz. protein

3 oz. cooked chicken or shrimp
16 oz. can chinese vegetables
4 oz. sliced mushrooms
1 pkg. Sweet 'N Low
3 T. soy sauce
1 garlic clove, crushed

In pan, mix all ingredients and simmer 10 minutes.

Tuna Omelet
Serves 3
1 serving = 4 oz. protein

3 eggs
1½ T. skim milk
dash salt
⅛ t. dill weed
4 oz. white tuna in water, drained
1 oz. grated cheese

Mix in a blender first 4 ingredients. Scramble egg mixture in pan over low heat. As eggs begin to set, add tuna and cover with grated cheese. Remove from heat and cover until cheese melts.

Pizza Pie
Serves 1
1 serving = 4 oz. protein, 1 milk, 1 slice bread

Crust:
1 egg

1 slice bread
⅓ cup dry milk
¼ t. baking powder
dash garlic powder

Beat egg and bread, stir in remaining ingredients. Spray baking dish with Pam and spread dough and bake at 400° for 10 minutes. Use Slim-U tomato sauce on top of pizza crust and top with 1 oz. mozzarella cheese and fresh sliced mushrooms.

Tuna Melt
Serves 4
1 serving = 4 oz. protein, ¼ milk

3 eggs
1 (7 oz.) can water packed tuna, drained
3 oz. shredded cheese
4 oz. mushrooms, sliced
1 cup skim milk
½ t. salt
dash paprika

Mix all ingredients together and place in a 9-inch pie plate. Bake at 350° for 45 minutes.

Seafood Cakes
Serves 2
1 serving = 6 oz. protein, ⅛ cup milk

10 oz. chopped shrimp, lobster or crabmeat
1 egg
2 T. parsley
1 T. dill seed
¼ t. curry
salt and pepper
powdered milk

Combine all ingredients *except* milk and form into patties. Coat these with powdered milk. Broil until brown.

Clam Chowder
Serves 1
1 serving = 6 oz. protein, 4 oz. *number 4* vegetable, 8 oz. tomato juice

2 oz. carrots
2 oz. peas
8 oz. French style string beans
1 envelope instant bouillon
1 cup tomato juice
1 T. green pepper, chopped
pinch of oregano
1 small can minced clams and juice

Combine in saucepan all ingredients *except* clams and simmer for 5–10 minutes. Add clams and juice just before serving.

Zucchini Omelet
Serves 1
1 serving = 4 oz. protein

2 eggs
zucchini
1 T. parmesan cheese
salt and pepper

Spray pan with Pam. Brown zucchini and season with salt and pepper. Add beaten eggs and cheese. Cook.

Asparagus Quiche
Serves 4
1 serving = 4 oz. protein, ¼ cup milk

1 can (10½ oz.) cut asparagus, drained
1 cup skim milk
4 eggs
1 small onion, finely minced
¼ lb. swiss cheese, shredded
½ t. leaf basil
1 t. salt
⅛ t. pepper

Place asparagus spears in bottom of 9-inch pie plate. Beat milk and eggs in medium size bowl; add remaining ingredients. Bake at 325° for 30 minutes or until knife inserted one inch from edge comes out clean.

Tuna or Turkey and Swiss Pita
Serves 4
1 serving = 4 oz. protein, 1 bread

8 t. mustard
4 small pita breads
8 oz. turkey or tuna
4 oz. swiss cheese, sliced

Heat oven to 350°. Spread mustard on the inside of each pita. Fill with turkey or tuna and cheese and wrap each sandwich loosely with aluminum foil. Bake 15 minutes, until cheese melts.

Casserole a la Zucchini
Serves 1
1 serving = 4 oz. protein, 6 oz. tomato juice

1 zucchini, cut in cubes
1 cup mushrooms
1 egg beaten
6 oz. tomato juice
¼ t. garlic powder
¼ t. parsley
1 t. onion flakes
1 t. celery flakes
1 oz. grated cheese

Spray pan with Pam. Cook zucchini and mushrooms until tender. Add egg, stir in tomato juice and seasonings. Put in baking dish and top with cheese. Bake at 375° for 30 minutes.

Teriyaki Steak
Serves 1
1 serving = 6 oz. protein

⅛ cup soy sauce
1 small garlic clove
½ cup warm water
2 packets Sweet 'N Low
2 (3 oz.) pieces lean rib eye of beef

Put meat in shallow dish and cover with all ingredients. Marinate for 2 hours. Broil.

Teriyaki Steak
Serves 2
1 serving = 6 oz. protein, 1 oz, *number 4* vegetable

1 cup tomato juice, cooked down
1 T. soy sauce
dash garlic powder
1 t. onion, chopped
dash worcestershire sauce

1 clove garlic, minced
½ cup mushrooms, sliced
1 lb. lean and trimmed London broil

Mix first 7 ingredients together. Use to marinate london broil over night. Broil.

Beefburgers
Serves 4
1 serving = 6 oz. protein

1 cup thinly sliced onion
2 lbs. lean ground beef or veal, shaped into burgers
¼ t. salt
pepper to taste
¼ cup beef broth

Brown onions, stirring frequently. Sprinkle burgers with salt and pepper. Add to onions. Cook through, remove burgers, keep warm. Drain grease and add beef broth, stirring constantly. Return burgers and cook 1 minutes, basting with sauce.

Stir-Fried Beef and Zucchini
Serves 4
1 serving = 4 oz. protein, 2 oz. *number 4* vegetable

⅓ cup water
2 T. soy sauce
1 pkg. Sweet 'N Low
1 t. salt
dash oil
1 large onion, sliced
2 medium zucchini, sliced diagonally
1 lb. lean ground round, chuck, or veal
1 can (8 oz.) sliced bamboo shoots, drained

1. Combine water, soy sauce, sweetener and salt.
2. Add oil, onion and zucchini. Stir-fry until vegetables are tender-crisp. Remove with a slotted spoon.
3. Add beef; stir-fry over high heat until well browned. Restir soy sauce mixture; add to beef. Return vegetables to pan; add bamboo shoots; stir-fry until heated. Spoon onto platter.

Veal Scallopini
Serves 4
1 serving = 6 oz. protein

1½ lbs. veal round steak, cut ½-inch thick
1 t. salt
dash pepper
1 cup mushrooms
½ cup water
1 T. lemon juice
¼ t. rosemary or tarragon or marjoram

Cut veal into 4 serving pieces. Sprinkle with salt and pepper. Spray pan with Pam and brown veal steaks. Add mushrooms, water, lemon juice and rosemary. Simmer covered for 10 minutes.

Broiled Meat Loaf
Serves 3
1 serving = 6 oz. protein, 1 oz. bread

1 lb. lean ground beef or veal
3 slices bread, toasted and crushed
1 egg
½ cup chopped parsley
½ t. chopped garlic
1½ T. water
½ t. salt
¼ t. ground cumin
½ t. oregano

Mix all ingredients together. Place in loaf pan. Bake at 350°
for 45 minutes.

Quick Franks
Serves 2
1 serving = 6 oz. protein, 4 oz. *number 4* vegetable

    1 large onion, sliced
    1 can (16 oz.) stewed tomatoes, cut up
    1 T. chili powder
    ½ t. salt
    1 lb. frankfurters

In medium skillet, saute onion until tender. Add tomatoes,
chili powder and salt; cover and simmer 10 minutes. Add
frankfurters; heat.

Stuffed Peppers
Serves 4
1 serving = 6 oz. protein, 1 oz. *number 4* vegetable

    8 green peppers
    2 lbs. lean ground beef or veal
    6 oz. tomato juice
    1 egg
    1 onion, chopped
    1 T. instant beef broth
    dash pepper
    dash garlic powder
    dash oregano

Clean out peppers. Mix veal or beef, egg, onion, pepper,
garlic, oregano, beef broth and 2 oz. tomato juice. Fill
peppers. Place in baking dish, pour remaining tomato juice
over peppers. Cover and bake at 350° for 1 hour.

Franks and Rice
Serves 2
1 serving = 1½ oz. protein, 4 oz. *number 4* vegetable

> 1 envelope bouillon
> ½ cup water
> ¼ cup onion, chopped
> ¼ cup celery, chopped
> 1 green pepper, chopped
> 4 oz. tomato sauce
> 1 can bean sprouts, drained
> ¼ t. garlic powder
> 1 t. buttered salt
> ¼ t. pepper
> ⅛ t. thyme
> 1 bay leaf
> 12 oz. frankfurters

In frying pan, dissolve bouillon in water. Add remaining ingredients and simmer covered for 30 minutes. Add frankfurters, cover and simmer an additional 15 minutes.

Meatballs
Serves 3
1 serving = 6 oz. protein, 4 oz. *number 4* vegetable

> 1 egg
> 1 lb. lean ground beef or veal
> 1 onion, chopped
> 1 t. dry mustard
> ¼ t. oregano
> 1 t. Sweet 'N Low
> salt and pepper to taste

Mix all ingredients together and form into balls. In saucepan combine: ¼ cup soy sauce, ½ cup tomato juice, and 1 teaspoon Sweet 'N Low. Add meatballs and simmer covered for 30 minutes.

Steak Kabobs
Serves 2
1 serving = 6 oz. protein

1 lb. cubed sirloin
button mushrooms
green pepper squares
onion chunks
salt and pepper to taste

Arrange meat and vegetables on skewers and broil 10–15 minutes, turning often. Season with salt and pepper.

Veal Rolls
Serves 2
1 serving = 8 oz. protein, 4 oz. *number 4* vegetable

1 lb. veal scallopini
salt and pepper
1 cup tomato juice
½ cup beef bouillon
½ onion, sliced
½ carrot, in strips

Season veal with salt and pepper. Wrap veal around vegetables and secure with a toothpick. Brown rolls in beef bouillon. Add tomato juice and cook slowly for 1 hour.

Veal Stew
Serves 4
1 serving = 6 oz. protein, 4 oz. *number 4* vegetable

2 lbs. veal, cubed
1 small onion, peeled

4 cups carrots, cut
salt and pepper to taste
2 bay leaves
2 cups water
2 T. wine vinegar
1 T. onion, chopped

Brown meat add onion, vinegar, bay leaves, salt, pepper, onion, and water. Simmer covered 1½ hours. Add carrots and simmer ½ hour more.

Veal á La
Serves 2
1 serving = 6 oz. protein

½ green pepper, diced
¼ pound mushrooms
½ cup skimmed milk
½ cup stock
¼ cup diced pimento
salt and pepper
12 oz. cut-up cooked veal

Cook pepper and mushrooms in a hot dry skillet for about 5 minutes, turning constantly. Add milk, stock, pimento, and seasonings, and cool gently, stirring constantly. Just before serving, add veal and heat it up but do not let it boil.

Pumpkin Loaf Cake
Serves 4
1 serving = 1 oz. number 4 vegetable, ¼ slice bread, 1½ oz. protein, 8 oz. milk, ¼ fruit

½ cup canned pumpkin
1 slice white bread
2 eggs
⅔ cup powdered milk (dry)
4 packets sweetener
½ t. baking soda
¼ t. cream of tartar
½ t. butter extract (optional)
½ t. coconut extract or almond extract

Put all ingredients in blender and turn on and off until well blended. Bake in small loaf pan sprayed with Pam, at 350° for about 40 minutes.

Topping

4 oz. riccota cheese
1 pkg. Sweet 'N Low
½ t. coconut extract
½ cup crushed pineapple

Mix all together and spread on cooled cake.

Custard
Serves 4
1 serving = 2 oz. milk, 1 oz. protein

1 cup skim milk
1 egg
2 pkgs. Sweet 'N Low
½ t. vanilla
pinch salt
cinnamon

Mix all ingredients together except cinnamon. Pour into baking dish or individual custard dishes and sprinkle with cinnamon. Set dish in pan of water and bake at 325° for 1 hour.

Cinnamon Crisps
Serves 7
1 serving = 1 bread all

15 slices melba diet bread
½ cup water
¼ t. cinnamon
4 packets Sweet 'N Low

Cut diet bread into 4 squares each. Prepare a solution of water, Sweet 'N Low, and cinnamon. Dip each square into the sweetened solution and place on Pam-sprayed or non-stick baking sheet. Place in a 350° oven and watch carefully as they crisp, turning if necessary.

Fruit Shake
Serves 1
1 serving = 1 fruit, 1 milk

½ cup cold water
2 small peaches, pitted, sliced
⅓ cup nonfat dry milk
2 large ice cubes

Place all ingredients in blender. Cover and blend at high speed for 30 seconds.

Cheeseless Cheesecake
Serves 4
1 serving = 1 milk, 1 fruit

Make in blender:
    1 (20 oz.) can crushed pineapple in its own juice
    2 pkgs. unflavored gelatin
    2 pkgs. Sweet 'N Low
    ½ cup boiling water
Blend for 2 minutes and add:
    2 t. lemon juice
    2 t. vanilla extract
    *1½ t. butter extract
    1 pkg. instant milk or enough of any powdered
        milk to make a quart

Blend for 2 minutes, pour into a 10-inch pie dish and sprinkle with cinnamon. Chill.

*For chocolate cake substitute 1 teaspoon chocolate extract for butter.

Lemon-Lime Chiffon
Serves 6
1 serving = 1 oz. protein

3 eggs, separated
1½ cups water, divided
¼ cup Sweet 'N Low
1 pkg. lemon gelatin
¼ cup lime juice
½ t. each grated lemon and lime peel
Whipped topping
lemon and/or lime slices (optional)

In small saucepan mix egg yolks, 1 cup water and ¼ cup Sweet 'N Low, stir over low heat until mixture comes to a boil and is thickened; remove from heat. Stir in gelatin until dissolved, then stir in remaining ½ cup water, the lime juice and peels. Chill until the consistency of unbeaten egg whites. Beat until stiff peaks form. Fold in gelatin mixture. Chill until firm, about 4 hours. Garnish with whipped topping and lemon and lime slices.

Baked Pears or Apples
Serves 4
1 serving = 1 fruit

4 pears or apples
1 can diet soda (black cherry, lemon, etc.)
1 t. cinnamon
1 pkg. Sweet 'N Low

Wash and core pears or apples. Place in baking dish. Pour diet soda over pears, sprinkle Sweet 'N Low and cinnamon on top. Bake at 350° for 1 hour.

Fluffy Limes
Serves 2
1 serving = 1 milk

1 cup evaporated skim milk
2 T. lime juice
green food coloring, 3 or 4 drops
4 pkgs. Sweet 'N Low
1 t. unflavored gelatin

Combine gelatin and Sweet 'N Low in pan and add milk. Stir over low heat until gelatin dissolves. Add coloring and chill in freezer until thick. Whip with mixer until stiff while adding lime juice. Beat until fluffy. Serve within 2 hours.

Strawberry Whip
Serves 4
1 serving = 1 fruit, ½ cup skim milk

½ cup evaporated skim milk
2 cups fresh or frozen strawberries
2 egg whites
2 pkgs. Sweet 'N Low
6 berries for garnish

Pour skim milk into small metal pan. Freeze until ice crystals form around edge of pan, approximately 30 minutes. Put strawberries into blender cover and blend until smooth. In small bowl beat egg whites until stiff. Fold berry puree into egg whites. Whip chilled milk until foamy. Add sweetener and continue beating until thick and fluffy. Fold in strawberry mixture. Pour into 4 parfait glasses. Serve immediately or refrigerate for 1 hour.

Almond Peach Pudding
Serves 4
1 serving = 4 oz. milk, ½ oz. protein, ½ fruit

2 cups skim milk
2 eggs
1 pkg. Sweet 'N Low
½ t. almond extract
½ t. cinnamon
½ t. nutmeg
2 peaches sliced fine

Mix first 6 ingredients in blender, fold in peaches. Pour into baking dish. Place baking dish into larger dish with an inch of water on bottom. Bake for 1 hour at 350°.

Pineapple Frosty
Serves 5
1 serving = 1 fruit

1 (20 oz.) can crushed pineapple
3 T. frozen orange juice concentrate

Mix in container with cover. Snap on cover and freeze until mixture is frosty cold.

Lemon Jello
Unlimited

¼ cup lemon juice
7 pkgs. Sweet 'N Low
pinch salt
1 cup hot water
1 cup cold water
1 packet unflavored gelatin

Soften gelatin in cold water, add hot water stirring until dissolved. Add remaining ingredients. Chill till firm.

French Pear Pudding
Serves 4
1 serving = 1 fruit, ¼ cup milk, ½ oz. protein

4 pears, peeled, halved and cored
½ cup strawberry jelly
1 cup skim milk
1 egg
1 pkg. Sweet 'N Low
1 t. vanilla
dash cinnamon and nutmeg

Beat together with milk, egg twin, vanilla, cinnamon, and nutmeg. Place pears in baking dish, pour custard mixture over pears. Place baking dish in a pan of water, bake at 325° for 1 hour. When cool spread jelly over top.

Lemon Custard
Serves 2
1 serving = ½ egg, ¼ cup milk

1 egg
2 packages Sweet 'N Low
⅛ t. salt
½ cup skim milk
2 t. lemon juice

Mix all ingredients. Pour into 2 custard cups. Set cups in pan of *hot* water. Bake at 350° for 45–60 minutes. Cool before serving.

Mock Rice Pudding
Serves 1
1 serving = 4 oz. protein, 1 bread, 1 fruit

3 oz. cottage cheese
1 egg
1 slice bread
½ cup crushed pineapple, in its own juice
1 t. imitation butter flavoring
1 t. vanilla
2 pkgs. Sweet 'N Low
dash cinnamon and nutmeg

Beat egg, break up bread and add to egg. Add remaining ingredients except cinnamon and nutmeg. Pour into baking dish, sprinkle with cinnamon and nutmeg, and bake at 350° for 30 minutes.

Fluff
Serves 4
1 serving = 1 glass of milk

Prepare jello according to package directions. Chill. Remove from refrigerator and add 1 tablespoon of dry skim milk. Beat with beater. Return to refrigerator.

Cream Cheese Pie
Serves 4
1 serving = 4 oz. protein

18 oz. cottage cheese
½ t. nutmeg
¼ t. cinnamon
½ t. rum flavoring
½ t. vanilla
1½ t. liquid sugar substitute
2 eggs, separated

Beat all ingredients except egg whites at high speed in electric blender with rotary beater until smooth. Do not underbeat. Fold in stiffly beaten egg whites. Place in a 7-inch pie pan. Set on botton shelf of broiler rack. Broil 8 minutes or until top is brown. Serve hot, or even better, cold. Sliced strawberries may be placed on top just before serving, but remember to count them as fruit.

Baked Pineapple
Serves 4
1 serving = 1 fruit

1 fresh pineapple, sliced
1 can low calorie cherry soda

Place pineapple and soda in a baking dish and bake at 350° for 45 minutes.

Holiday Fruit Pudding
Serves 4
1 serving = 1 fruit, 1 bread

3 apples, peeled, and diced
1 t. cinnamon
2 T. grated orange peel
3 T. brown Sugar Twin
4 slices bread, cubed
1 t. lemon juice
1 cup blueberries
1 cup water

Combine all ingredients in a mixing bowl, mix well. Turn into a 1 quart casserole and bake at 400° for 45 minutes.

Quick Fruit Cup
Serves 6
1 serving = 1 fruit

1 cup cantaloupe balls
1 can pineapple tidbits (in own juice)
½ cup juice from canned pineapple

½ cup orange juice
2 T. lemon juice

Drain pineapple, reserve liquid. Combine pineapple juice with orange and lemon juice. Add fruit juice to melon balls and pineapple. Chill thoroughly before serving.

Nothings
Serves 2
1 serving = 1 cup milk, 2 eggs

4 egg whites
1 t. vanilla extract
1 t. almond extract
4 pkgs. Sweet 'N Low
⅔ cup dry milk
cinnamon

Beat egg whites until stiff. Fold in dry milk and mix well. Add extracts and Sweet 'N Low. Spoon drop on a cookie sheet and bake at 275° for 45 minutes. Remove from sheet and dust with cinnamon.

Apple Ice
Serves 2
1 serving = 1 fruit

½ cup water
6 T. frozen apple juice concentrate

Blend in blender to mix. Add 8–10 ice cubes one at a time and blend until the consistency of snow.

Apple Deliteful
Serves 1
1 serving = 1 fruit, 4 oz. protein, 1 bread all

1 T. unflavored gelatin
1 medium apple, peeled, cored, and sliced
1½ cups diet cream soda
1 t. cinnamon
2 pkgs. Sweet 'N Low
⅔ cup riccota cheese
½ t. vanilla
1 slice white bread, crumbled

In saucepan bring soda to a boil. Remove from heat; sprinkle gelatin over soda. Stir until dissolved. Refrigerate until mixture is syrupy. Place half of apple slices in baking dish. Combine cinnamon and Sweet 'N Low and sprinkle ¼ of the mixture over the apples. Spoon half of the gelatin mixture on top. Mix riccota cheese, half of the cinnamon–Sweet 'N Low mixture and vanilla extract. Spread over apple slices. Sprinkle bread over cheese mixture. Arrange remaining apple slices and cinnamon–Sweet 'N Low mixture over bread. Spoon remaining gelatin over top. Bake at 325° (slow oven) for 1 hour. Serve chilled.

Apple Tarts
Serves 6
1 serving = ½ slice bread, ½ fruit

3 apples
1 t. lemon juice
1 T. diet margarine
cinnamon and Sweet 'N Low to taste
2 slices bread

Peel the apples, slice and place in small pan with a little water and lemon juice. Cook just until soft (comstock apple pie slices unsweetened may be used). Add Sweet 'N Low and cinnamon to taste. Put into Pam sprayed tart forms. Toast two slices regular bread and crumble in blender. To toast crumbs add 1 tablespoon diet margarine, cinnamon and 2 pkgs Sweet 'N Low. Sprinkle crumbs over tarts. Artificial brown sugar may be sprinkled over tarts for extra sweetness.

Applesauce Squares
Serves 4
1 serving = 1 slice bread, ½ tablespoon margarine, 1 fruit

4 slices bread, toasted and made into crumbs
¼ t. cinnamon
¼ t. nutmeg
1 pkg. Sweet 'N Low
2 T. melted diet margarine
2 cups applesauce
2 T. lemon juice
1 shredded lemon rind

Preheat oven to 350°. Mix together bread crumbs, cinnamon, nutmeg and margarine. Spray baking dish (8-inch) with Pam, press ⅔ of this mixture into dish. Combine applesauce, twin, lemon juice and rind. Pour into baking dish and top with remaining crumbs. Bake for 30 minutes.

Apple Supreme
Serves 4
1 serving = 1 fruit, 1 bread, 1 oz. protein, ½ milk

4 slices very thin bread
4 pkgs. Sweet 'N Low
2 eggs
2 cups nonfat dry milk
½ t. baking soda

½ t. baking powder
1 T. butter flavoring
¼ t. salt
½ t. lemon peel

Mix all ingredients together. Spray square pan with Pam and pour ingredients into pan.

Place in sauce pan:
4 apples, peeled and sliced
1 T. lemon juice
1 T. water
1 t. cinnamon
¼ t. nutmeg
4 pkgs. Sweet 'N Low

Cook covered for 5 minutes. Pour evenly over batter and sprinkle with cinnamon. Bake at 375° for 30 minutes.

Hippy Holidays:
Poetry to Lose Weight By

The most important thing to remember about a holiday is that it is the day before you start dieting.

My New Year's Resolution every year, of course is, "This year I am going to lose weight." Sound familiar? Most people make this toast with a three hundred and fifty calorie brandy Alexander in one hand and chip and dip in the other. In fact, you make a vow to join Slim-U right after the holidays are over.

Happy New Rear

New Year's Eve brings a tear to my eyes
Didn't stay on my diet, but gave many tries
For the last twelve months I ate like a pig
My stomach and can sure did get big

Here I stand in my basic black dress
The seams are giving way under stress
My bra straps are cutting my shoulders in two
And my girdle is turning my body bright blue

The top of the girdle has rolled and curled
I'm nervous, depressed, and ticked at the world
Next year I'll be thin and wear shocking pink
Now on with food and down with my drink!

For Lincoln's Birthday you buy a chocolate nut roll. Of course, you aren't going to eat any because you're going on a diet. Well, just a taste. Valentine's Day you buy your husband a large box of candy and help him eat it. Washington's Birthday you bake the family a deep-dish cherry pie—here's to the Father of our Country. St. Patrick's Day everyone is Irish, so everyone must eat corned beef and potatoes, washed down with beer. Erin Go Bragh.

March. If it weren't for Girl Scout Cookies and my company from up north I might be safe for a couple of weeks. But who can resist a Girl Scout? Of course we are one of the few people in the world who cherish the little things in life and observe the little holidays such as Ground Hog Day, Flag Day and Lassie's birthday. It's always hard to know what to serve on these days as there is no tradition to follow, but we always come up with something. United in brotherhood we stand. Passover and Easter, I'll eat bagels in your honor if you'll eat jelly beans to honor me.

Ode To Easter

Fat women buy Easter candy far in advance
The good stuff goes fast and they can't take a change

We look high and low to make our deposit
And find the best place is up in the closet

We think all day about that chocolate rabbit
And when nobody's home, we're bound to grab it

We'll wolf it down from tail to ear
Now eggs and jelly beans all disappear.

Mother's Day—that's me—Mom! The day I wait for all
year. Today I can do anything I want, it's my day so I'll eat,
eat, eat.

Mother's Day

M is for the mounds of food she's eaten
O is for the other crap she's chewed
T is for the tons of carbohydrates
H is for the hot dogs and booze
E is for the ever mounting fat cells
R is for the rounder that she got

Put them all together, they spell MOTHER
The fattest lady on our block.

Father's Day. That means Dad can do anything he wants
to do. I'll make him his favorite dinner and a two-layer
chocolate cake. If the truth be known, I'm the reason he gets
to celebrate, I'm the one who made him a father, so I'll eat,
eat, eat.

Father's Day

Father's Day is for Mother too
She did her part to bring about you

She'd be thin and cute if she had her way
But your old man wanted his Father's Day

She gained fifty pounds while carrying her son
And she can't seem to lose it, though you are forty-one

Though Father's Day is big in our nation
Mom can remember it was her ruination.

Fourth of July. The annual family picnic, and you know
how I love picnics! You folks just go ahead and shoot off your

fireworks, I'm going to clean the table and consolidate the salads. Of course, if I hadn't sneaked so much potato salad we wouldn't have to consolidate so often. August is rather a dull month for eating because there aren't any big holidays, but with a little luck and extensive research, you will probably be able to find a family birthday somewhere in the Family Bible to celebrate. I can remember one hot August, looking all through our illustrious family history, and finally coming up with two birthdays and the anniversary of a great uncle who was hanged as a horse thief. When you need an occasion, you need an occasion. So here's to Unkie. Thirty days hath September and a Labor Day Picnic. Oh thank Heaven!

October is a wonderful month. First there is my birthday.

Happy Birthday

I was eight and one-half-pounds when my birthdays began
I had round face and a large soft can
Then I added a year and a whole lot of weight
I was eating and gaining at a hell of a rate

In the snap of a finger sweet Barbara was five
And ate more at a meal than a whole pygmy tribe
The first day of school I walked like a duck
To find clothes to fit me was a sure stroke of luck

Sweet sixteen for a fat girl's not great
If you've spent all those years licking your plate
Twenty five birthdays have crept up on you
And your new birthday dress is a cute size twenty-two

Thirty-six candles, one to grow on makes seven
And the dial on your scales has now reached 211
Add the pounds to the years and it sure makes me blue
Happy Birthday Dear Fatass Happy Birthday to you!

Then Bilinda's birthday (cake) and then Halloween. Oh

happy day. First you get your child a large brown paper bag and help color spooky faces on it. Second, find a suitable costume because the sweeter they look, the more candy they'll get, and after all that's the name of the game. Third, send them out early, the good stuff goes fast. Be sure to send Daddy out with the kids, this way you can eat all the candy you want and blame it on the goblins. Fourth, upon your ballerina's return home, take the treat bag away immediately so you can check for suspicious goodies. This also gives you a chance to mentally sort out your own favorites. Fifth, gently put your tired, candy stuffed darling to bed and DIG IN. No guilt please, we are only trying to keep them from diabetes, pimples, bad teeth and fat.

Halloween

Fall was ending, winter coming,
    the season in between
The holiday all fat kids love,
    they call it Halloween

You carve your pumpkin way ahead
    and watch that sucker rot
The more the toothy mouth sunk in
    the sourer it got

You told yourself such spooky tales
    you were scared to get in bed
You remembered all those ghostly books
    that you had ever read

But one thing kept you going and
    looking straight ahead
It was all the goo and garbage that would
    turn your ass to lead

You looked and looked for weeks and weeks for
    just the right wrap
You found it and set right off to
    get your bag of crap

The first house gave a Hershey
  and you ate it right away
Fat kids never save a lick to
  eat another day

Remember how your fat legs ran to hit
  the place next door
No matter how much junk you ate there was
  always room for more

When you got home, your Mom was shocked
  to see the bag was clean
She knew damn well you ate it all,
  cause your fat little face was green!

Finally it's November—the beginning of the Holiday Season! Thanksgiving and fat people are more thankful than the average bear—thanks for the potatoes, gravy, stuffing, corn, hot rolls, nuts, creamed onions, and a special thanks for the pie.

Thanksgiving

Thanksgiving Day what a delight!
Thanksgiving Day, the greatest, it meant
We eat, eat, eat
What all year long's a no-no is now a legal treat
We eat all kinds of nibbles, fixing din-din
For the folks
We can sneak a lot of goodies
And hear those sick fat jokes
If things are going to turn out right
You know you'll have to taste
And the more you check for salt and spice
The thicker gets your waist
Potatoes, gravy, stuffing, corn
And see old chubs dig in
And everytime we chew, chew, chew
We grow another chin
The diet starts tomorrow
So have another piece of pie

I'm not sure what I'm thankful for
I think I'm going to die!

December—Hoorah—deck the halls, trim the tree and let's get on with the feast. Christmas and Hanukkah give unlimited opportunities to eat which prompted me to re-write this for my Slim-U groups.

'Twas the Night Before Christmas

'Twas the night before Christmas, no one was awake
'Cept a member of Slim-U looking for cake.
The stockings were hung by the chimney with care
And she knew that some goodies could be hidden there.
She once had been nestled all snug in her bed
But visions of sugarplums danced in her head.
So out she came in her old flannel wrap
And started her search for some kind of crap.
She looked in the cookie jar without any clatter
So the kids wouldn't come to see what was the matter.
She flew to the closet, her eyes really flashed
And looked with great love where the fruit cake was stashed.
The glaze on the cake gave a wonderful glow, candied fruit
And walnuts—"Oh, I love you so!"
When what to her wondering eyes should appear
But a big ripe banana—she ate without fear.
Then she ate another—Oh boy was she quick
'Cause she knew with that stomach she'd never get sick.
More rapid than eagles the courses they came,
Cause once you start eating it all tastes the same.
First grapes, now figs, and a handful of candy
You know once she's started she'll eat anything handy.
Tomorrow is Christmas and she will have a ball
And when nobody's looking she will eat it all.
As she threw back her head and was turning around
She saw her reflection and did her heart pound.
She was covered in fat from her head to her feet
What she saw in that mirror just wasn't too neat.
She looked ten years older because of the fat
And when she punched her stomach her stomach jumped
    back.

But her eyes how they twinkled, her dimples how merry
When she thought of a sundae topped with a cherry.
Her droll little mouth will draw up like a bow
When she thinks of the cheating that only she'd know
When she thinks of the junk she had passed through her teeth
Of course it was just to give her stomach relief.
She has a broad rear and a round little belly
That shakes when she laughs like a bowl full of jelly.
And soon she will say, "I'm ashamed of myself."
With a tear in her eye and her rear full of lead
Now she's decided to go back to bed.
Just to be slim is her Christmas wish
But back go the fingers in the old candy dish.
She crawled in her bed and heaved a big sigh
And promised tomorrow to pass up the pie.
To eat like a pig—she thinks is no sin
So her brain gives a shout
"Next year I'll get slim!"

Slim-U Menu Plans

As we've said many times, this isn't really a diet book, but we've got to face the facts here and realize that not everyone on the face of this earth is a Julia Child. So for those of you whose mind goes blank at menu planning when the chocolate soufflés and spaghetti and meat balls are taken off the menus, here's a month's worth of meals to start you on your way to being slim.*

*The asterisked recipes can be found in the Slim-U recipe section of this book. Check this section before you prepare any of these dishes!

Week One

Sunday

Breakfast
1 Scrambled Egg
1 Slice Toast
Diet Margarine
Peach Preserves*
Beverage

Lunch
Bean & Beef
  Salad*
Cheeseless
  Cheesecake*
Beverage

Dinner
Veal à La*
Broccoli Soufflé*
Lemon Lime
  Chiffon*

Monday

Breakfast
French Toast
Apple Butter*
Beverage

Lunch
Cream Cheese
  Pie*
Beverage
Quick Fruit Cup*

Dinner
Beefburgers*
Asparagus
Tossed Salad*
Lemon Custard*

Tuesday

Breakfast
1 Scrambled Egg
Toast with Peach
  Preserve*
Beverage

Lunch
Tuna Omelet*
Cinnamon
  Crisps*
Beverage

Dinner
Chicken Creole*
Summer Salad*
Veggie
  Potpourri*

Wednesday

Breakfast
Flategg Muffins
4 oz. Orange Juice
Beverage

Lunch
Tuna or Turkey
  and Swiss
  Pita*
Applesauce
  Squares*
Beverage

Dinner
Shrimp Scampi*
Asparagus
  Vinaigrette*
French Pear
  Pudding*
Beverage

Thursday

Breakfast
1 oz. Bran Cereal
  with Skim Milk
⅓ cup Cottage
  Cheese with
  Crushed
  Pineapple
Beverage

Lunch
Asparagus
  Quiche*
Beverage

Dinner
Chicken &
  Broccoli*
Cucumber and
  Onion Salad*
Holiday Fruit
  Pudding*
Beverage

Friday

Breakfast	*Lunch*	*Dinner*
Cantaloupe Ideal*	Apple Deliteful*	Quick Franks*
Beverage	Beverage	Braised Escarole
		& Tomatoes*
		Lemon Lime
		Chiffon*

Saturday

Breakfast	*Lunch*	*Dinner*
Breakfast	Broccoli Spread*	Stir-Fried Beef &
Sandwich*	with Raw	Zucchini*
Beverage	Vegetables	Garden Salad*
	Gelatin	Quick Fruit Cup*

Week Two

Sunday

Breakfast	*Lunch*	*Dinner*
1 Slice Toast	Cheese Omelet	Steak Kabobs*
Crushed Pineapple	Pineapple	Tossed Salad*
Grilled Cheese	Frosty*	Beets
Beverage		Almond Peach
		Pudding*

Monday

Breakfast	*Lunch*	*Dinner*
Jelly Roll*	Cheese &	Veal Stew*
4 oz. Orange Juice	Spinach	Cucumber
Beverage	Casserole*	Salad*
	Apple Tarts*	Quick Fruit Cup*

Tuesday

Breakfast	*Lunch*	*Dinner*
1 Egg	Pizza Pie*	Teriyaki Steak*
Toast	Tossed Salad*	Broccoli &
Apple Butter*	Beverage	Chestnuts*
Beverage		Cauliflower &
		Cheese
		Lemon Jello*

Wednesday

Breakfast
Apple Crumb
    Special*
Beverage

Lunch
Casserole à la
    Zucchini*
Baked Pear*
Beverage

Dinner
Franks & Rice*
Chocolate
    Cheeseless
    Cheesecake*

Thursday

Breakfast
Complete
    Breakfast*

Lunch
Clam Chowder*
Summer Salad*
Beverage

Dinner
Salmon Steak
String Beans &
    Mushrooms
Pumpkin Loaf*

Friday

Breakfast
Breakfast
    Sandwich*
Beverage

Lunch
Chicken Stuffed
    Tomato on
    Lettuce
Fluff*

Dinner
Shrimp
Broccoli with
    Cheese*
Chocolate
    Cheeseless
    Cheesecake*

Saturday

Breakfast
Omelet*
4 oz. Orange Juice
Beverage

Lunch
Seafood Cakes*
Custard*

Dinner
Tuna Casserole*
Tossed Salad*
Apple Tidbits*

Week Three

Sunday

Breakfast
Apple Muffins*
Beverage

Lunch
Mock Rice
    Pudding*
Gelatin
Beverage

Dinner
Japanese
    Chicken*
Tossed Salad*
Broccoli
Baked
    Pineapple*

Monday

Breakfast
Cantaloupe Ideal*
Beverage

Lunch
Broccoli Cheese
   Dish*
Beverage

Dinner
Scallop Sticks*
Tossed Salad*
Carrots
   Supreme*
Fluff*

Tuesday

Breakfast
4 oz. Orange Juice
½ Bagel with
  American Cheese
Beverage

Lunch
Spinach Salad*
Pineapple
   Frosty*

Dinner
Meatballs*
Cole Slaw
Asparagus
Custard*

Wednesday

Breakfast
½ Grapefruit
Poached Egg on
   Toast
Beverage

Lunch
Tuna Melt*
Apple Ice*
Tossed Salad*
Vinaigrette
   Dressing*

Dinner
Veal Rolls*
Cucumber
   Salad*
Apple Tidbits*

Thursday

Breakfast
Apple Tidbits*
   Leftovers
Beverage

Lunch
Enchilada*
Fruit Shake*

Dinner
Hurry-Up
   Chicken*
Baked Squash
   French Style*
Green Beans
Fluffy Limes*

Friday

Breakfast
1 Scrambled Egg
Toast, Peach
   Preserves*
Beverage

Lunch
Chef Salad
Vinaigrette
   Dressing*
Beverage
Almond Peach
   Pudding*

Dinner
Stuffed Peppers*
Chinese
   Vegetable
   Salad*
Cauliflower
Gelatin

Saturday

Breakfast	*Lunch*	*Dinner*
Pineapple	Quick Lunch*	Tuna Casserole*
Bread Pudding*	Tossed Salad*	Great Zucchini*
Beverage	Baked Pear*	Cucumber Salad*
		Strawberry Whip*

Week Four

Sunday

Breakfast	*Lunch*	*Dinner*
1 Scrambled Egg	Stuffed Tomatoes (Zucchini)*	Green Bean Chili*
Apple Supreme*	Cheeseless Cheesecake*	Pumpkin Loaf*
	Beverage	Beverage

Monday

Breakfast	*Lunch*	*Dinner*
½ Bagel	Orange Chicken Salad*	Broiled Meat Loaf*
Crushed Pineapple	Beverage	Herbed Green Peas*
Grilled Cheese		Tossed Salad*
Beverage		Lemon Custard*

Tuesday

Breakfast	*Lunch*	*Dinner*
1 Egg over Lightly on 1 Slice Thin Toast	Tuna Stuffed Tomatoes on Lettuce	Veal Scallopini*
4 oz. Orange Juice	Lemon Custard*	String Beans & Mushrooms
		Great Zucchini*
		Baked Apple*

Wednesay

Breakfast
French Toast with
   Diet Margarine
   & Diet Jelly
½ Grapefruit

Lunch
Orange Chicken
   Salad*
Beverage

Dinner
Teriyaki Steak*
Chinese
   Vegetable
   Salad*
Broccoli cooked
   with Boullion
Lemon Custard*

Thursday

Breakfast
Breakfast
   Sandwich*
Beverage

Lunch
Zucchini
   Omelet*
Tossed Salad*
Beverage

Dinner
Italian Scallops*
Asparagus
Carrots
Cheeseless
   Cheesecake*

Friday

Breakfast
1 Scrambled Egg
1 Piece Thin Toast
   with Margarine
4 oz. Orange Juice

Lunch
Pita Bread
   Sandwich—
   Bean Sprouts,
   Sliced Tomato
   & Cheese
Fresh Fruit Cup*
Beverage

Dinner
Mushroom
   Stuffed
   Chicken*
Vegetables Del
   Sol
Unsweetened
   Apple Sauce
Cheeseless
   Cheesecake*

Saturday

Breakfast
Pancakes*
4 oz. Orange Juice

Lunch
Zucchini
   Omelet*
Tossed Salad*
Beverage

Dinner
Shrimp & Pea
   Salad*
Pumpkin Loaf*
Beverage

Index